Herbs and Spices

Edited by Muhammad Akram and Rabia Shabir Ahmad

Published in London, United Kingdom

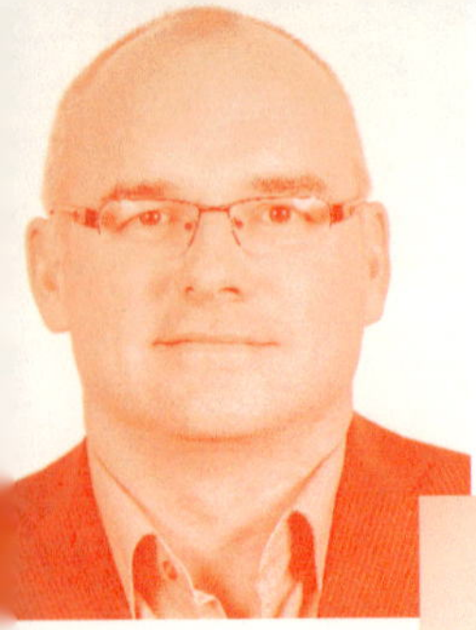
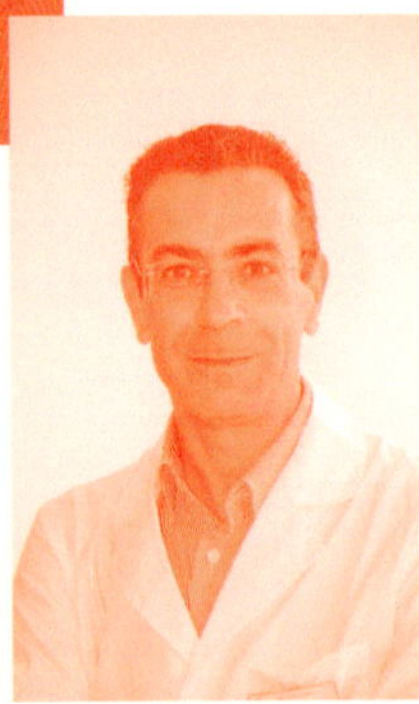
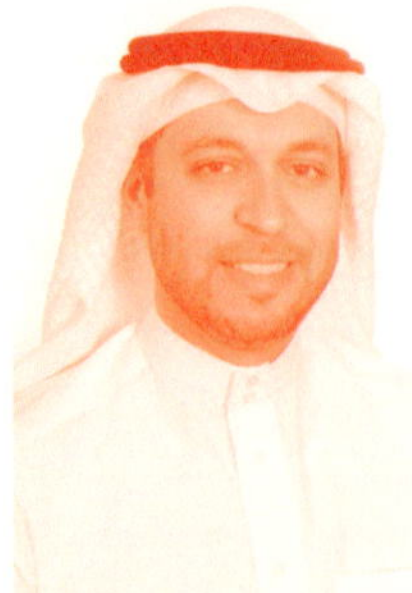
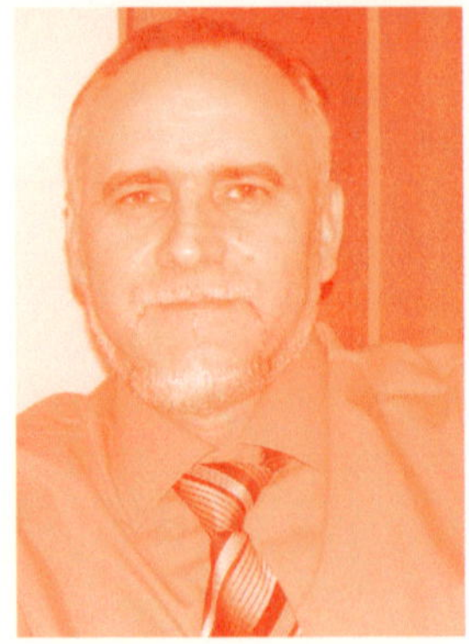
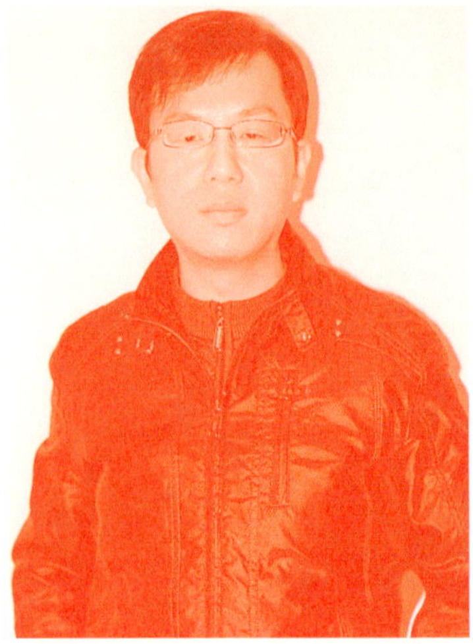
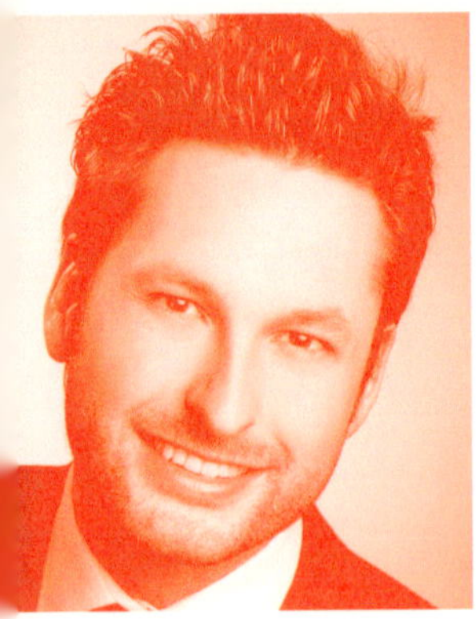
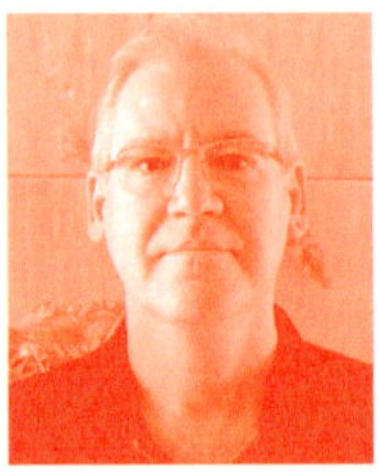

IntechOpen

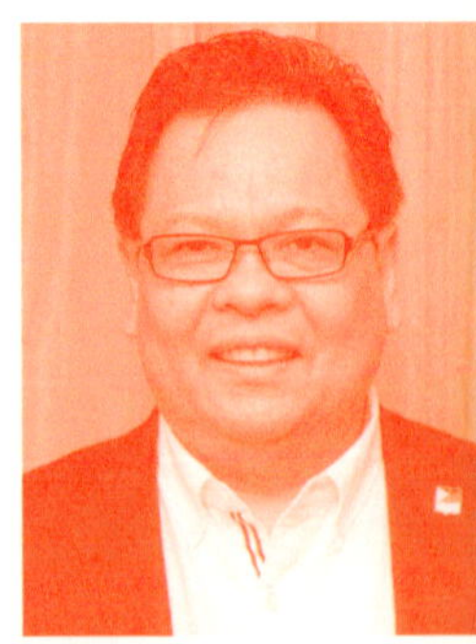
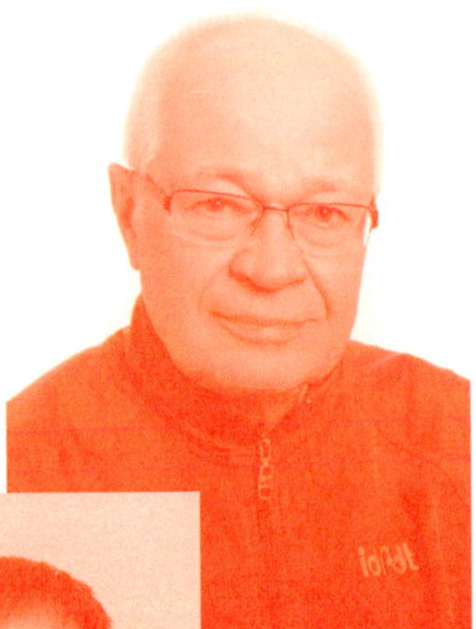
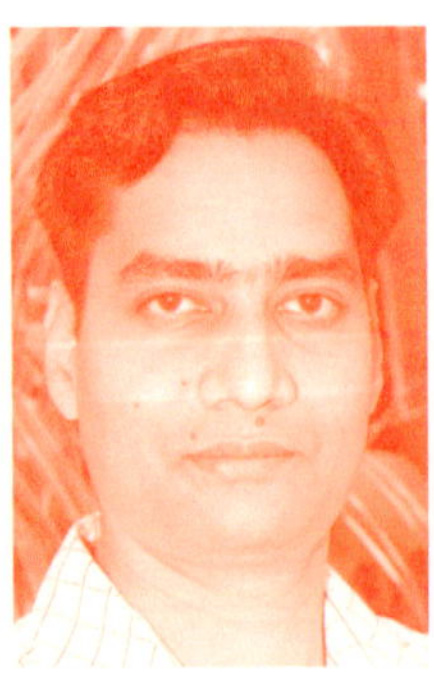
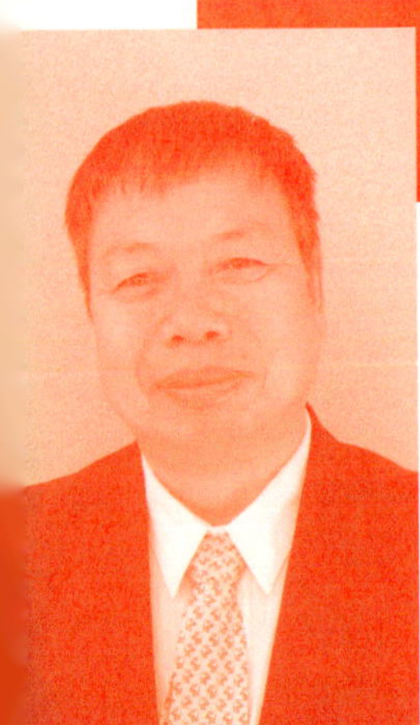
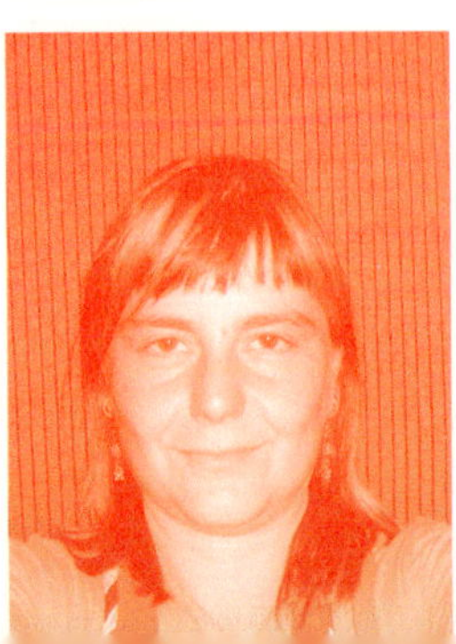
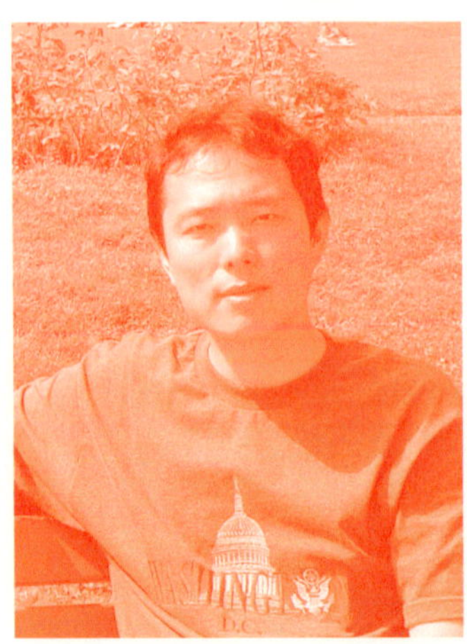

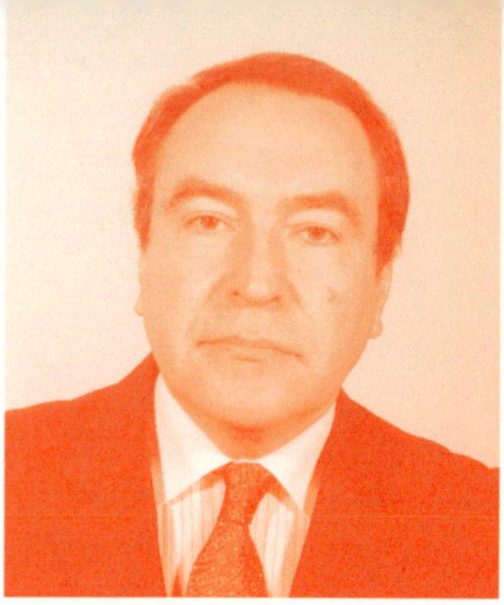

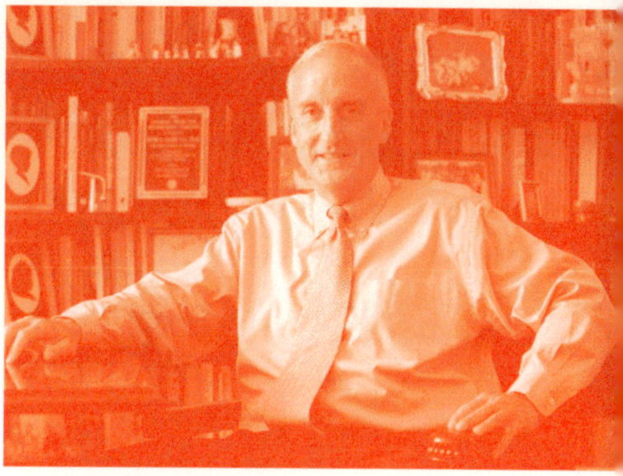

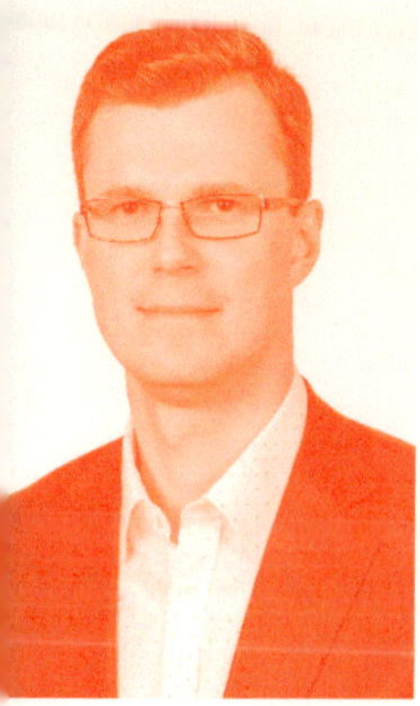

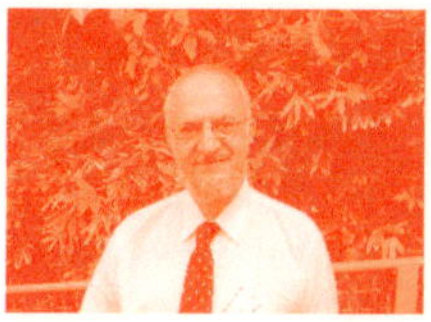

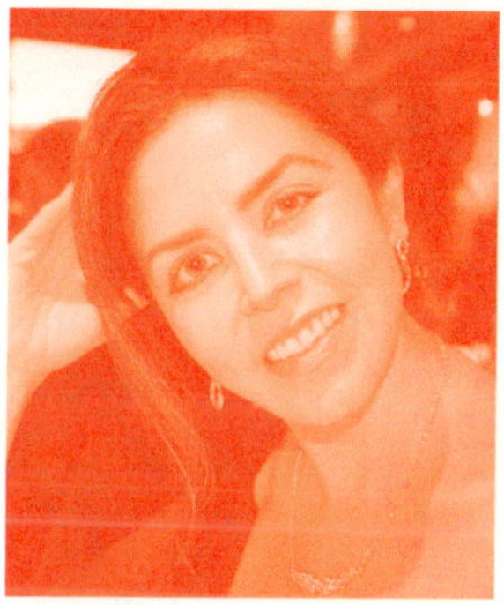

Supporting open minds since 2005

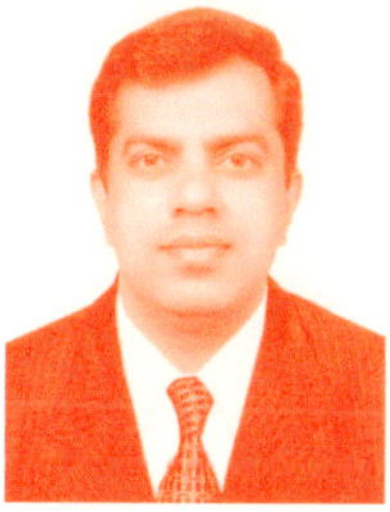

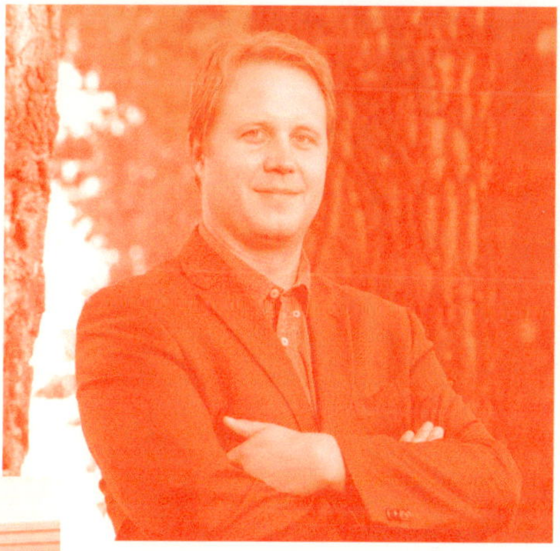

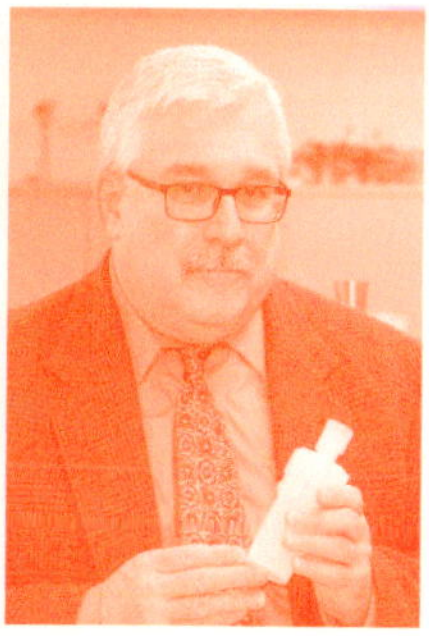

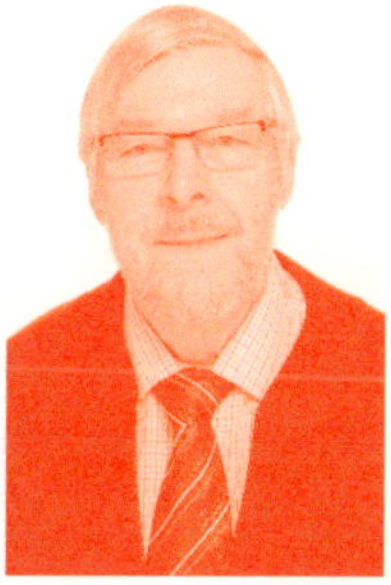

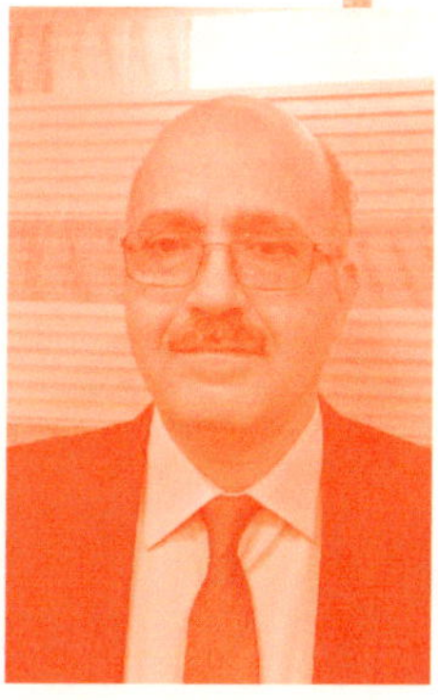

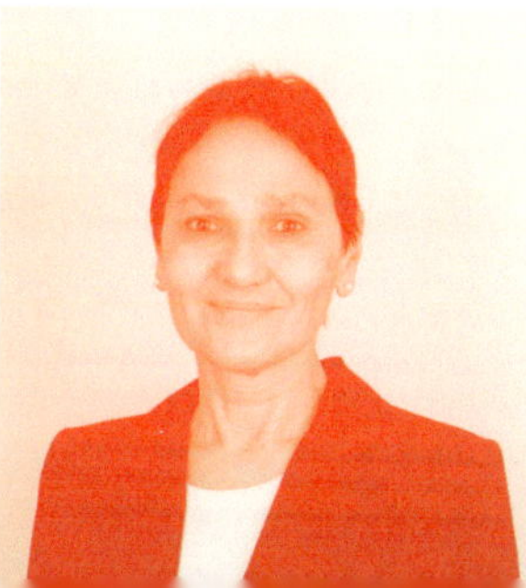

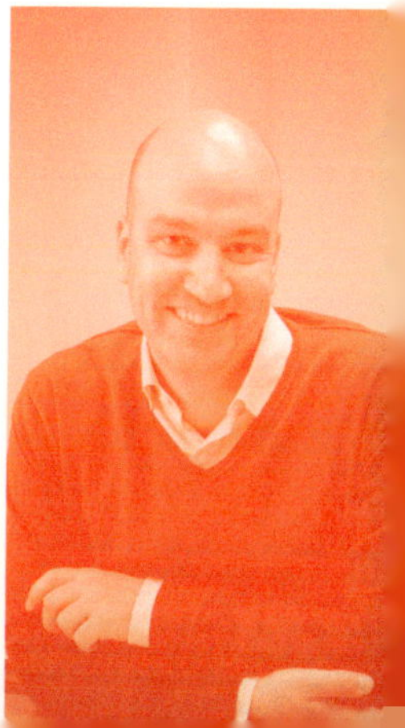

Herbs and Spices
http://dx.doi.org/10.5772/intechopen.73759
Edited by Muhammad Akram and Rabia Shabir Ahmad

Contributors
Sadeq Sabeeh Kareem Altaie, Noor Falah Mahde AL-Kenane, Yordan Martínez, Dairon Más, Thukaa Abdul-Jalil, Afaque Quraishi, Gyanmani Ekka, S.K. Jadhav, Naveen Kumar Dubey, Edziri Hayet, Rim Nasri, Marwa Hamdi, Maha Mastouri, Monique Mancuso, Rabia Shabir Ahmad, Ali Imran, Muhammad Sajid Arshad, Muhammad Bilal Hussain, Marwa Waheed, Saira Safdar, Zarina Yasmin

First published in London, United Kingdom, 2020 by IntechOpen
IntechOpen is the global imprint of INTECHOPEN LIMITED, registered in England and Wales, registration number: 11086078, 5 Princes Gate Court, London, SW7 2QJ, United Kingdom
Printed in Croatia

British Library Cataloguing-in-Publication Data
A catalogue record for this book is available from the British Library

Additional hard and PDF copies can be obtained from orders@intechopen.com

Herbs and Spices
Edited by Muhammad Akram and Rabia Shabir Ahmad
p. cm.
Print ISBN 978-1-83962-935-8
Online ISBN 978-1-83962-936-5
eBook (PDF) ISBN 978-1-83962-937-2

For EU product safety concerns:
IN TECH d.o.o., Prolaz Marije Krucifikse Kozulić 3, 51000 Rijeka, Croatia,
info@intechopen.com or visit our website at intechopen.com.

Meet the editors

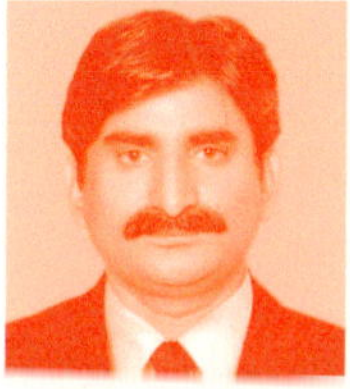

Muhammad Akram is currently working as the Chairperson and Associate Professor at the Government College University Faisalabad, Pakistan. He obtained his PhD degree in Eastern Medicine from Humdard University, Pakistan. He is serving as an Mphil and PhD supervisor. He has published 151 journal papers, 11 books, and 10 book chapters. He has attended national and international conferences as speaker. He is currently serving as a reviewer and editorial board member of multiple reputed high impact factor journals. His research interests include: phytochemistry, bioactivity, and phytopharmaceutical evaluation of herbs, medicinal plants, biochemistry and bioinformatics. Currently, he is serving as a potential member of national and international scientific committees.

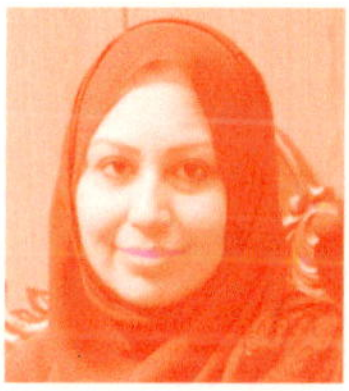

Dr. Rabia Shabir Ahmad has a strong academic, teaching, and research background. She has a number of credits and honors in her career. The academic career of Dr. Rabia Shabir is comprises brilliant successes. In every competitive environment, she has proved herself the best. During her academic carrier, she secured a merit scholarship from the University of Agriculture, Faisalabad for her Bachelors and Masters degrees. She received a PhD Indigenous Scholarship during her PhD. Dr. Rabia Shabir Ahmad played an important role in the establishment and development of the Institute of Home and Food Science at GC University, Faisalabad. She developed and taught courses to graduate and post-graduate level students both in food science and technology and human nutrition and dietetics. During her stay at the Government College University Faisalabad, she won various HEC Funded research projects and she was also honored to receive the highest funded project under the NRPU scheme from HEC. Along with her teaching and research supervising responsibilities, she has also been working as the reviewer of several journals. She has published numerous research papers in highly impacted international and national journals. She is active in developing laboratories and laid the strong foundation of research at the Institute of Home and Food Sciences.

Contents

Preface XI

Chapter 1 1
Introductory Chapter: *Mentha piperita* (a Valuable Herb): Brief Overview
by Rabia Shabir Ahmad, Ali Imran, Muhammad Sajid Arshad, Muhammad Bilal Hussain, Marwa Waheed, Saira Safdar and Zarina Yasmin

Chapter 2 11
Role of Herbs and Medicinal Spices as Modulators of Gut Microbiota
by Yordan Martínez and Dairon Más

Chapter 3 27
Study Biochemistry of *Mentha longifolia* (L.) Huds.: A Review
by Sadeq Saheeh Kareem Al-Taie and Noor Falah Mahde Al-Kenane

Chapter 4 39
Rhus coriaria (Sumac): A Magical Spice
by Thukaa Zuhair Abdul-Jalil

Chapter 5 53
An Overview of Genus *Zanthoxylum* with Special Reference to Its Herbal Significance and Application
by Gyanmani Ekka, Shailesh Kumar Jadhav and Afaque Quraishi

Chapter 6 71
Metabolomics
by Naveen Kumar Dubey

Chapter 7 83
The Antibacterial Activity of *Mentha*
by Monique Mancuso

Chapter 8 93
Determination of In Vitro Antiprotease, Antimicrobial, and Antibiofilm Activities of *Beta vulgaris* var. cicla against Multidrug-Resistant Strains of *Pseudomonas aeruginosa*
by Hayet Edziri, Rim Nasri, Marwa Hamdi and Maha Mastouri

Preface

This edited volume is a collection of reviewed and relevant research chapters concerning the latest developments within the agricultural and biological sciences fields of study. The book includes scholarly contributions by various authors and has been edited by a group of agricultural and biological experts.

Each contribution comes as a separate chapter, complete in itself but directly related to the book's topics and objectives.

There are 8 chapters in this book and they are as follows:

CHAPTER 1: Introductory Chapter: *Mentha piperita* (a Valuable Herb): A Brief Overview

CHAPTER 2: Role of Herbs and Medicinal Spices as Modulators of Gut Microbiota

CHAPTER 3: Study Biochemistry of *Mentha longifolia* (L.) Huds.: A Review

CHAPTER 4: *Rhus coriaria* (Sumac): A Magical Spice

CHAPTER 5: An Overview of Genus *Zanthoxylum* with Special Reference to its Herbal Significance and Application

CHAPTER 6: Metabolomics

CHAPTER 7: The Antibacterial Activity of *Mentha*

CHAPTER 8: Determination of In Vitro Antiprotease, Antimicrobial, and Antibiofilm Activities of *Beta vulgaris var. cicla* against Multidrug-Resistant Strains of *Pseudomonas aeruginosa*

The target audience comprises scholars and specialists in the agricultural and biological sciences fields.

IntechOpen

Chapter 1

Introductory Chapter: *Mentha piperita* (a Valuable Herb): Brief Overview

Rabia Shabir Ahmad, Ali Imran, Muhammad Sajid Arshad, Muhammad Bilal Hussain, Marwa Waheed, Saira Safdar and Zarina Yasmin

1. Introduction

In different parts of the world, herbs were utilized for medicines, food, and many other purposes. In various countries, research is being done to discover the potential applications of medicinal plants in favor of human beings [1]. *Mentha* was described and named by Jussieu in 1789. It is a member of the Lamiaceae family, and their plants generally contain flowers with prominent liplike lower petals. Small trees, perennial or annual herbs, and shrubs are members of this family. The genus *Mentha* has been in a state of flux with especial reference to its taxonomy, as more than 3000 names have been being published since 1753. Keeping in view the chromosome numbers, phylogenetic analysis, and major essential oil components, *Mentha* has been redefined to comprise of 18 species and 11 hybrids, which are divided into four sections [2]. These species are herbaceous and perennial plants, commonly cultivated for flavor and a pleasant aroma. Natural menthol has a soothing and relaxing cooling impact on the mucous membrane of the human body and on the skin. Oil extracted from *Mentha* has cosmetic, pharmaceutical, and perfumery applications. Sometimes, it is also used for culinary purposes for food and flavors [3].

2. Classification

Kingdom: Plantae plants
Phylum: Magnoliophyta
Class: Magnoliopsida
Order: Lamiales
Family: Lamiaceae
Genus: *Mentha*
Species: Piperita [4]

3. Cultivation

Mints have the potential to grow nears water pools, rivers, lakes, and partially moist cool spots. They also can grow under the sun. These can grow throughout the year [5]. For its cultivation, Mediterranean Basin is a primary resource, but tropical and temperate regions are mostly noted as the best resource. *Mentha* is not cultivated in South America and Antarctica. But in all other countries, it is widely distributed. Australia, Europe, Central Asia, and North Africa are the main centers of the genus *Mentha* cultivation [6].

4. Description

Mints are the aromatic and perennial herbs, having overground and underground stolons, which are quite widespread. They also have square, erect, and branched stems. The arrangement of their leaves is in opposite pairs, from oblong to lanceolate with the downy approach and sharp edges. The color profile of *Mentha* leaves is quite broad ranging from blue, dark green, grayish green to purple, and it could be pale yellow. *Mentha* flowers are being produced in false whorls also known as verticillasters, and their color range is from white to purple. A flower having two-lipped corolla portion with four lobes and its fruit has 1–4 seeds, covered with a stony layer [2].

5. Species

The following is a list of some major species of Mentha used for medicinal purpose (**Table 1**).

5.1 *Mentha arvensis*

Mentha arvensis is an aromatic branched herb that can reach a height of 40 cm, with terminal branches in ascending position. Leaves are 1.5–2 cm in length, round-tipped with tooted margins having the shape of oblong-ovate. The flowers produced

S.N.	Species name	Function	Picture	Reference
1	*Mentha arvensis* L.	The plant is used to treat liver and spleen diseases, asthma, and jaundice	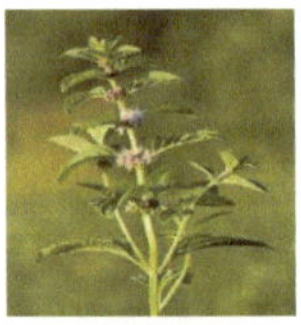	[7]
2	*Mentha longif olia* (L.) L.—horsemint	Longifolia L. is used as a medicinal plant with properties including antispasmodic, antimicrobial, anti-bloating, anti-coughing, and antiasthmatic	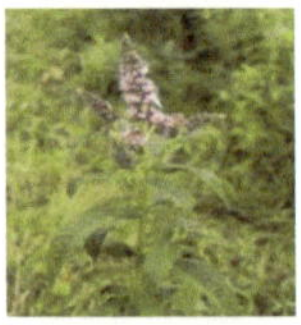	[8]
3	*Mentha puleg ium* L.—pennyroyal	Pennyroyal is frequently used as an insecticide and pest repellent	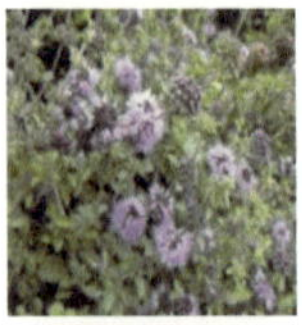	[9]
4	*Mentha aquatica*	Mint was originally used as a medicinal herb to treat stomachache and chest pains, and it is commonly used in the form of tea as a home remedy to stimulate digestion	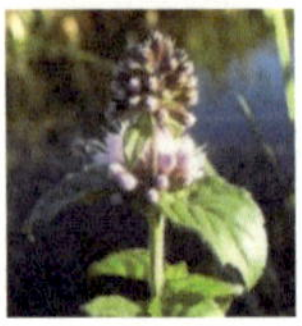	[10]

Table 1.
Major species of Mentha *plant used for medical purpose.*

on this plant are purplish to light blue in color, having hairs on them. It is used to cure the maladies of asthma, liver, jaundice, and spleen. Oil is procured from the distillation of leaves having 40–50% of menthol. Its oil is carminative, stimulant, antiseptic, and diuretic. Menthol is being used in drugs for the cure of stomach issues and in ointments for the remedy of headache. Its leaves are also deployed as a remedy for rheumatic pains and indigestion. Its active constituents comprise of menthone, menthol, limonene, methyl acetate, isomenthone, beta-caryophyllene, tannins, neomenthol, alpha- and beta-pinene, flavonoids, and piperitone. Its oil consists of 4.5–10% esters, menthyl acetate along with ketones with a percentage of 15–20% [11].

Mentha arvensis produces 70–90% of menthol along with cineol piperitone, sesquiterpene, and cineol piperitone as the other ingredients. The plant of mint contains chrysoeriol, eriocitrin, isorhoifolin, hesperidoside, methyl rosmarinate, linarin, narirutin, acacetin, tilicine, hesperidin, rutin, menthoside, luteolin, nodifloretin, and flavonoids diosmin. It also consists of the phenolic acids including lithospermic acid, protocatechuic acid, rosmarinic acid, daucosterol, β-sitosterol, anthraquinones aloe-emodin, phytosterols, chrysophanol, protocatechuic aldehyde, tannins, emodin, and caffeic acid [12] (**Figure 1**).

5.2 *Mentha longifolia* (L.) L.—horsemint

Mentha longifolia also called the horsemint; it is a native plant of Europe but not of Ireland and Britain. It is also present in the central and western Asia and in the northern and southern Africa. It is a herbaceous perennial plant having an aroma of peppermint. It includes rhizome having a creeping nature, which can grow up to a height of 40–120 cm. Its leaves are 5–10 cm long, 1.5–3.0 cm in width having above the color of green to grayish green with white color on the below side of leaves. Its flowers are of purple or white color, having a length of 3–5 cm in length, and are produced in thick clusters on branched and tall spikes. They produce flowers from mid to late summer, which form clonal colonies. They help in the cure of bad breath and protection of teeth. They also help in the removal of dandruff when used in combination with vinegar [13] (**Figure 2**).

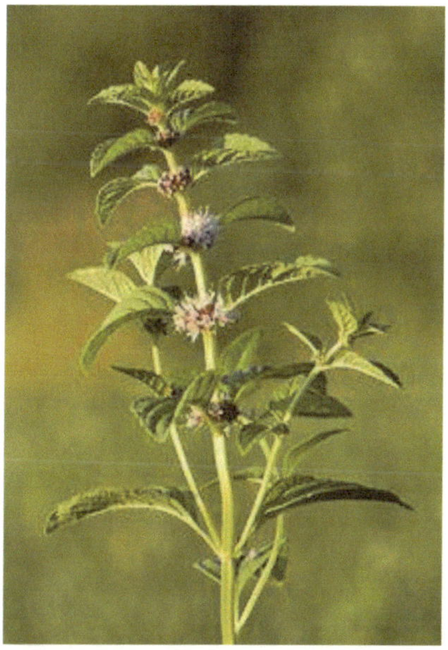

Figure 1.
Mentha arvensis *[7]*.

6.3 Room fragrance and aromatherapy

In ancient times, peppermint was known as the herb of kindness and warmth, and it was the first herb used in Europe as a room deodorizer. To diminish the smell of soil, the floor was covered with a sprinkled herb which spread its sweet scent throughout the room. Nowadays, because of the essential oil, peppermint is used for aromatherapy [22].

7. Unfavorable and toxic effect

There are several adverse side effects regarding peppermint. Peppermint and its major chemical components like menthone, menthol, pulegone, and menthofuran are proved to be toxic with a moderate effect on some individuals. Its essential oil combines with the cytochrome P450 isoenzyme in the liver microsomes of humans. The use of peppermint is restricted or must be used with caution in patients having inflammation in gall bladder and blockage of bile duct [23] (**Table 2**).

S. N.	Species Name	Function	Picture	Reference
1	*Mentha suaveolens*	*Mentha suaveolens* is used for medicinal purposes for thousands of years in many parts of the world, including Africa, Europe, Asia, and the Americas	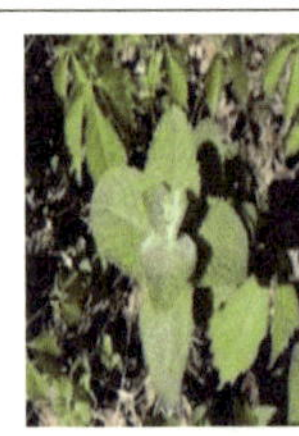	[24]
2	Peppermint	A common side effect of the oral intake of peppermint oil or capsules is heartburn. Oral use of peppermint products may have adverse effects when used with iron supplements, cyclosporine, medicines for heart conditions or high blood pressure, or medicines to decrease stomach acid	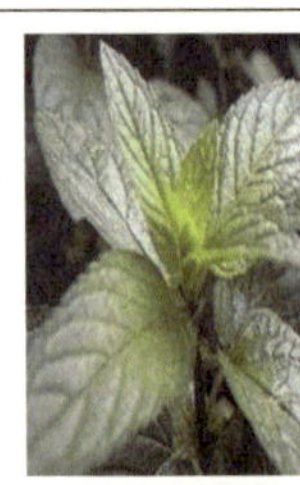	[10]
3	*Mentha requienii*	In traditional medicine, this plant has been used as an antiseptic, a carminative, and a febrifuge The smell of mint is disliked by rats and mice, and this plant has been used for strewing on the floor to deter rodents	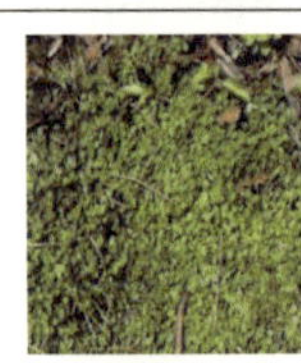	[25]
4	Spearmint	It is used as a flavoring for toothpaste and confectionery and is sometimes added to shampoos and soaps	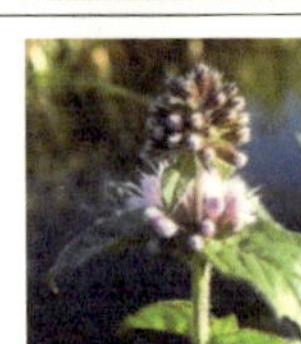	[26]
5	*Mentha canadensis*	It is grown in Hungary for essential oil and menthol production	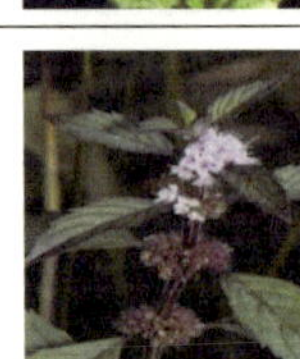	[27]

S. N.	Species Name	Function	Picture	Reference
6	*Mentha australis*	It is used as bush food, an insect repellent, and is also said to have medicinal properties. *Mentha australis* is commonly called River Mint	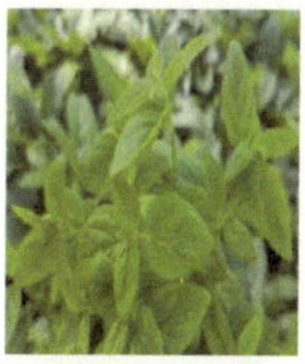	[28]
7	*Menthe gracilis*	It is used as the traditional flavoring of Scotch mint candies. In Vietnamese cuisine, the fresh herb is used as a flavoring in chicken or beef. As a medicinal herb, it is used to treat fevers, headaches, and digestive ailments	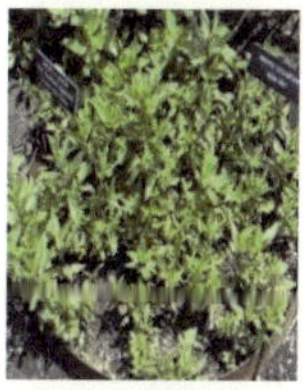	[29]
8	*Mentha dahurica*	It is used as a culinary herb and medicinal herb. It is used as a groundcover	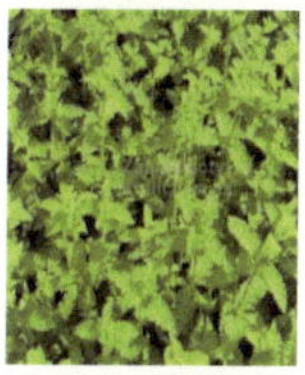	[30]
9	*Mentha diemenica*	The plant was therefore used in homes as a strewing herb and has also been spread in granaries to keep the rodents off the grain	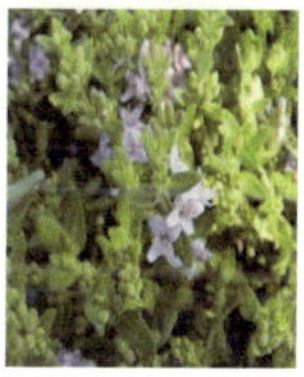	[31]

Table 2.
Other well-known species of Mentha *plant used for medical purpose.*

Acknowledgements

The authors are highly obliged to the Library Department, Government College University Faisalabad, Pakistan and IT department, Higher Education Commission (HEC, Islamabad) for access to journals, books and valuable database.

Conflict of interest

The authors declare no conflict of interest.

Author details

Rabia Shabir Ahmad[1*], Ali Imran[2], Muhammad Sajid Arshad[1], Muhammad Bilal Hussain[2], Marwa Waheed[2], Saira Safdar[1] and Zarina Yasmin[3]

1 Department of Food Science, Nutrition and Home Economics, Faculty of Life Sciences, Government College University, Faisalabad, Pakistan

2 Institute of Home and Food Sciences, Faculty of Life Sciences, Government College University, Faisalabad, Pakistan

3 Post Harvest Research Centre, Ayub Agriculture Research Institute, Faisalabad, Pakistan

*Address all correspondence to: rabiaahmad@gcuf.edu.pk

References

[1] Heinrichs PA, Nikolaus CJ, Ellison B, Nickols-Richardson SM, Chapman-Novakofski K. Vegetables, herbs and spices: The importance of family and tasting. Health. 2016;**8**(14):1554

[2] Lawrence BM. Mint: The Genus *Mentha*. Boca Raton, FL, USA: CRC Press; 2006

[3] Ansari MA, Vasudevan P, Tandon M, Razdan RK. Larvicidal and mosquito repellent action of peppermint (*Mentha piperita*) oil. Bioresource Technology. 2000;**71**(3):267-271

[4] Kanakis CD, Petrakis EA, Kimbaris AC, Pappas C, Tarantilis PA, Polissiou MG. Classification of Greek *Mentha pulegium* L. (pennyroyal) samples, according to geographical location by Fourier transform infrared spectroscopy. Phytochemical Analysis. 2012 Jan;**23**(1):34-43

[5] Taneja SC, Chandra S. Mint. In: Handbook of Herbs and Spices. Sawston, UK: Woodhead Publishing; 2012. pp. 366-387

[6] Salehi B, Stojanović-Radić Z, Matejić J, Sharopov F, Antolak H, Kręgiel D, et al. Plants of genus *Mentha*: From farm to food factory. Plants. 2018; 7(3):70

[7] Akram M, Uzair M, Malik NS, Mahmood A, Sarwer N, Madni A, et al. *Mentha arvensis* Linn.: A review article. Journal of Medicinal Plant Research. 2011;**5**(18):4499-4503

[8] Mikaili P, Mojaverrostami S, Moloudizargari M, Aghajanshakeri S. Pharmacological and therapeutic effects of *Mentha longifolia* L. and its main constituent, menthol. Ancient Science of Life. 2013;**33**(2):131

[9] Aziz EE, Rezk AI, Omer EA, Nofal OA, Salama ZA, Fouad H, et al. Chemical composition of *Mentha pulegium* L. (pennyroyal) plant as influenced by foliar application of different sources of zinc. Egyptian Pharmaceutical Journal. 2019;**18**(1):53

[10] McKay DL, Blumberg JB. A review of the bioactivity and potential health benefits of peppermint tea (*Mentha piperita* L.). Phytotherapy Research: An International Journal Devoted to Pharmacological and Toxicological Evaluation of Natural Product Derivatives. 2006;**20**(8):619-633

[11] Anwar F, Abbas A, Mehmood T, Gilani AH, Rehman NU. *Mentha*: A genus rich in vital nutra-pharmaceuticals—A review. Phytotherapy Research. 2019;**33**(10): 2548-2570

[12] Thawkar BS. Phytochemical and pharmacological review of *Mentha arvensis*. International Journal of Green Pharmacy (IJGP). 2016;**10**(2):71-72

[13] Farzaei MH, Bahramsoltani R, Ghobadi A, Farzaei F, Najafi F. Pharmacological activity of *Mentha longifolia* and its phytoconstituents. Journal of Traditional Chinese Medicine. 2017;**37**(5):710-720

[14] Goodarzi M, Nanekarani S. Effects of feeding *Mentha pulegium* L. as an alternative to antibiotics on performance of broilers. APCBEE Procedia. 2014;**8**:53-58

[15] Motamedi H, Seyyednejad M, Dehghani F, Hasannejad Z. Investigation of antibacterial activity of ethanolic and methanolic extracts of *Mentha pulegium* L. Zahedan Journal of Research in Medical Sciences. 2014; **16**(10):55-59

[16] Ashu Agbor M, Naidoo S. Ethnomedicinal plants used by traditional healers to treat oral health

problems in Cameroon. Evidence-Based Complementary and Alternative Medicine. 2015;**1**:2015

[17] Singh P, Pandey AK. Prospective of essential oils of the genus Mentha as biopesticides: A review. Frontiers in Plant Science. 2018;**9**:1295

[18] Fifi AC, Axelrod CH, Chakraborty P, Saps M. Herbs and spices in the treatment of functional gastrointestinal disorders: A review of clinical trials. Nutrients. 2018;**10**(11): 1715

[19] Carvalho IT, Estevinho BN, Santos L. Application of microencapsulated essential oils in cosmetic and personal healthcare products—A review. International Journal of Cosmetic Science. 2016;**38**(2): 109-119

[20] Hines S, Steels E, Chang A, Gibbons K. Aromatherapy for treatment of postoperative nausea and vomiting. Cochrane Database of Systematic Reviews. 2018;**3**:1-78

[21] Rodriguez-Fragoso L, Reyes-Esparza J, Burchiel SW, Herrera-Ruiz D, Torres E. Risks and benefits of commonly used herbal medicines in Mexico. Toxicology and Applied Pharmacology. 2008;**227**(1):125-135

[22] Sowndhararajan K, Kim S. Influence of fragrances on human psychophysiological activity: With special reference to human electroencephalographic response. Scientia Pharmaceutica. 2016;**84**(4): 724-751

[23] Malekmohammad K, Rafieian-Kopaei M, Sardari S, Sewell RD. Toxicological effects of Mentha x piperita (peppermint): A review. Toxin Reviews. 2019;**1**:1-5

[24] Božović M, Pirolli A, Ragno R. *Mentha suaveolens* Ehrh.(Lamiaceae) essential oil and its main constituent piperitenone oxide: Biological activities and chemistry. Molecules. 2015 May;**20** (5):8605-8633

[25] Chessa M, Sias A, Piana A, Mangano GS, Petretto GL, Masia MD, et al. Chemical composition and antibacterial activity of the essential oil from *Mentha requienii* Bentham. Natural Product Research. 2013;**27**(2):93-99

[26] Bimakr M, Rahman RA, Taip FS, Ganjloo A, Salleh LM, Selamat J, et al. Comparison of different extraction methods for the extraction of major bioactive flavonoid compounds from spearmint (*Mentha spicata* L.) leaves. Food and Bioproducts Processing. 2011; **89**(1):67-72

[27] Tucker AO, Chambers HL. *Mentha canadensis* L.(Lamiaceae): A relict amphidiploid from the lower tertiary. Taxon. 2002;**51**(4):703-718

[28] Tang KS, Konczak I, Zhao J. Identification and quantification of phenolics in Australian native mint (*Mentha australis* R. Br.). Food Chemistry. 2016;**192**:698-705

[29] Paulus D, Becker D, Nava GA, Luckmann D, de Andrade Moura C. Cultivation of mint (Mentha x gracilis) in intercropping with fruit trees in an agroforestry system: Production and quality of essential oil. European Journal of Medicinal Plants. 2019;**9**:1-9

[30] Zhang Y, Wang X, Miao T, Wang C. Research on the diversity of *Mentha dahurica* Fisch. Ex Benth. Of the Xiaoxing'an mountains area in Heilongjiang province. In: IOP Conference Series: Earth and Environmental Science. Vol. 358, No. 2. IOP Publishing; 2019. pp. 1-4

[31] Abbaszadeh B, Valadabadi SA, Farahani HA, Darvishi HH. Studying of essential oil variations in leaves of *Mentha* species. African Journal of Plant Science. 2009;**3**(10):217-221

Chapter 2

Role of Herbs and Medicinal Spices as Modulators of Gut Microbiota

Yordan Martínez and Dairon Más

Abstract

Currently, herbs, medicinal spices, green medicine, or traditional Chinese medicine has gained many followers in the world, especially as a way of life and as an alternative to the indiscriminate use of synthetic medicines such as antibiotics. These natural products are rich in secondary metabolites or phytochemicals, which are chemical compounds of relatively complex structures and restricted distribution; these compounds have defensive functions against insects, bacteria, fungi, parasites, and viruses. Likewise, several studies have shown their effectiveness in the prevention and treatment of several diseases such as cancer, autoimmune diseases, gastrointestinal diseases, diabetes, neurodegenerative diseases, Crohn's disease, and human immunodeficiency virus (HIV), among others. In addition, this review addresses the mechanisms of action of the herbs and medicinal spices on intestinal microbiota, increasing competitive exclusion in the intestinal membrane and inhibiting bacterial translocation and damage to the intestinal barrier.

Keywords: beneficial, diet, gut microbiota, health, phytochemical compound

1. Introduction

Through history, the individual and collective experiences of a population have been systematized and transformed as part of their popular culture, their means of action, and their wisdom. Popular customs based on empirical bases have found justification with the development of science and technology, after having been used for a long time. In this sense, due to advances in the areas of knowledge, especially medicine, genetics, immunology, and molecular biology, it is obvious to seek explanations and incontestable facts that justify the use of some popular practices that may be useful in the treatment of different health problems. These practices are phytochemical compounds, which have been the subject of deep research around the world [1].

The phytochemicals have been used for over 60,000 years to prevent or cure diseases that affect humans [2]. It is estimated that about 260,000 species of plants are known today, of which 10% can be considered as medicinal, with many phytochemical properties. According to the classification of medical treatments of phytotherapy, in modern and past times, many regions are favored by the proportion of phytochemical compounds, which can vary appreciably to the established percentage, since the totality of the vegetal flora is not known [3].

Despite the agro-industrial development of humanity and the strong influence of the large pharmaceutical industries, phytochemical compounds are the first sources for medical treatment in many countries, due to its effectiveness against different pathologies, low production cost, and slight residual effect [4–6]. Its use is strengthened and expanded more and more, appearing in new and novel active principles, both for human and veterinary use. It is estimated that between 75 and 80% of the world population used phytochemical compounds one way or another, China and India being the countries that used the natural products of plant origin the most, as part of their cultural roots. These beneficial phytobiotics are used mainly as food or part of the food, although they are also used as pharmaceutical preparations. In these countries, traditional medicine is used daily as a lifestyle to prevent, cure, and/or alleviate diseases. In this sense, natural compounds have been used to treat diseases that damage the nervous, cardiovascular, respiratory, gastrointestinal, renal, metabolic, immune, and musculoskeletal systems, besides preventing or curing metabolic disorders of the main biomolecules of the organism [7, 8].

Plants are natural laboratories where a large amount of chemical substances are biosynthesized, and in fact, they are considered the most important source of chemical compounds that exists. A large percentage of the active ingredients included are called "phytochemical compounds or secondary metabolites," which are chemical compounds of relatively complex structures and restricted distribution; among these metabolites, those with defensive functions against insects, bacteria, and fungi, among others, as alkaloids, non-protein amino acids, steroids, phenols, flavonoids, glycosides, coumarins, quinones, tannins, and terpenoids, are common. There is great variation in the concentration of these phytochemicals in the plant, and there is no maximum production pattern nor special storage organs; however, it is common that the highest concentrations of these types of compounds are in flowers, leaves, and seeds [9, 10].

Currently, research on natural products is focused on the discovery of new active ingredients with beneficial properties against several systemic and infectious diseases in humans and animals [11]. It has been proven that synthetic substances sometimes have more harmful side effects than the diseases they treat; some synthetic antioxidant compounds cause toxic and mutagenic effects [12]. Thus, several authors indicate the need to reuse natural preparations as alternatives to the indiscriminate use of antibiotics and their microbial resistance [13, 14]. However, it is currently unclear how phytochemical compounds have a high compatibility with the human organism [14], because these have no enzymatic affinity and are poorly absorbed by the intestinal lumen.

Intestinal microbiota plays an important role in maintaining intestinal integrity and function; a loss in microbial balance causes severe damage at the local and systemic level [15–17]. It is important to note that the microbiota in the first years of life of children is unstable, dominated mainly by *Clostridium leptum* and *Clostridium coccoides* species [18]. The phyla *Firmicutes*, *Bacteroidetes*, and *Actinobacteria* are dominant in the microbiota of healthy adults [19]. *Actinobacteria*, especially *Bifidobacteriaceae*, are found in small concentrations compared to the species belonging to the phylum *Firmicutes* and *Bacteroidetes*; however, they are very important as modulators of intestinal barrier function [20]. The phytochemical compounds may favor the growth of specific beneficial bacteria in the intestine under health or host disease conditions [21, 22].

Many investigations have focused on demonstrating the antimicrobial effect of phytochemical compounds; however, there are contradictions in the mechanism of action of the active principles. These phytochemicals compounds could have bacteriostatic or bactericidal action as well as inhibit the adhesion of pathogenic bacteria to the intestinal and urinary mucosa. Every day the use of phytochemicals to reduce the pathogenic effect of intestinal bacteria is more frequent, due to the increase of antimicrobial resistance to antibiotics [23, 24]. Therefore, the aim of this review is to summarize the role of herbs and medicinal spices like modulators of gut microbiota.

2. What are the phytochemical compounds?

Phytochemicals are chemical compounds synthesized by plants that fulfill nonessential functions, so that their absence is not fatal for it, since they do not intervene in the primary metabolism. These compounds intervene in the ecological interactions between the plant and its environment [25]. They also differ from the primary metabolites in that each of them has a restricted distribution in the plant kingdom, sometimes to only one species or a group of them, so many of them are useful in *Systematic Botany* [10]. For many years, the adaptive value of the most secondary metabolites was unknown. Many times, they were described as final products of metabolic processes, without a specific function, or directly as waste products of plants. In general, in the past they have received little attention by biologists and botanists, so many of the functions of secondary metabolites are still unknown [26].

The study of these substances was initiated by organic chemists of the nineteenth century and the beginning of the twentieth century, who were interested in these substances due to their importance as medicinal drugs, poisons, flavorings, glues, oils, waxes, and other materials used in the industry [27]. In fact, the study of phytochemicals stimulated the development of separation techniques, spectroscopy to elucidate their structure, and synthesis methodologies that today contribute to the development of contemporary organic chemistry [28].

In addition, the content of the active principles of a plant can vary significantly due to differences from one locality to another and, even within the same locality due to several agrochemical properties of the land, the season and variations for temperature, precipitation, pollution, lunar cycle, or other factors [5]. The plants have characteristics that allow them to influence through their components not only by direct contact but also remotely by means of emanations. There are plants that through the emanations of their active ingredients can eliminate the spores of fungi, protozoa, and malignant bacteria [2, 10]. The recognition of biological properties of many phytochemical compounds has encouraged the development of this field, for example, in the search for new drugs, antibiotics, insecticides, and herbicides. Moreover, the growing appreciation of the highly diverse biological effects of these compounds has led to the reevaluation of the different roles they have in plants, especially in the context of ecological interactions [10].

Phytochemicals can be divided into three large groups, based on their biosynthetic origins: phenolic compounds, terpenoids, and nitrogen compounds or alkaloids. They can also be divided according to their biosynthetic pathway and chemical structure: terpenoids, alkaloids, betalains, glucosinolates, cyanogenic glycosides, polyacetylenes, anthocyanins, and other flavonoids [26].

Currently, many synthetic drugs produced by the pharmaceutical industry have very harmful side effects and are not effective in alleviating or reducing the symptoms of many diseases such as cancer, HIV, Alzheimer's, and other chronic diseases. Therefore, modern medicines where phytochemicals are included as an alternative source may meet the therapeutic requirements of patients. In this sense, there is high availability of these natural products from plant sources that act as potent curative medicines [29]. Phytochemicals including polyphenols, flavonoids, and others have the potential to provide a defense against oxidative damage. Plant extracts and phytoconstituents are found to be effective as radical scavengers and inhibitors of lipid peroxidation [30, 31]. A wide range of antioxidants from both natural and synthetic origin to treat various human diseases has been proposed [32].

Other metabolites have wide medicinal properties, such as sterols used as part of hormones and vitamins; triterpenes have anthelminthic, antiseptic, expectorant, antibacterial, and diuretic activity. Simple phenols have antifungal activity. The tannins (condensed tannins) have astringent, antiseptic, antibacterial, and antifungal properties. The coumarins are used in medicine for their anticoagulant and antibacterial action. The flavonoid glycosides (anthocyanins and quercetins) are attributed effects on the blood supply of the bronchi and bronchodilation. Quinones (specifically naphthoquinones) are characterized by their antibacterial and antifungal action. Cardiotonic glycosides stimulate cardiac function. The alkaloids stimulate the central nervous system and have an anesthetic effect. Saponins are precursors of steroidal hormones and corticosteroids and have emulsifying and hemolyzing functions [4–6, 33].

3. Role of the phytochemical compounds to modulate gut microbiota

The gut microbiota begins to mature from the second year of life and has various roles such as nutrient absorption and food fermentation [34], proper modulation of the immune system to the gastrointestinal tract (GIT) of the host [35], and the physiological mechanisms against pathogens [36]. In adults, the most prevalent phyla representatives are *Bacteroidetes* and *Firmicutes*, *Clostridium leptum* and *Clostridium coccoides* being the dominant groups and *Lactobacillus* the subdominant in *Firmicutes* phyla [18, 19], a gut microbiota that is highly stable [37]. It is estimated that the gastrointestinal tract inhabits 500–1000 different microbial species, with the highest concentrations in the colon (up to 10^{12} cells per gram of feces); also, the presence of *E. coli* (in 7.7 log10 CFU/g) is considered a subdominant population in adults and dominant species in infants [38].

The bacterial population of the *Bifidobacterium* genus are minor constituents of the gut microbiota, whose concentration is eight to ten times lower than the two main phyla [39]. *Bifidobacterium* spp. enhance the barrier function of the gut epithelium and gut health; however, a decrease of the population of this bacterial genus causes chronic low-grade inflammation with lipopolysaccharide (LPS) (endotoxemia), related to multiple abnormal processes in the organism [40, 41]. Also, the composition of the microbiota in elderly individuals is affected by a significant reduction of *Bacteroidetes* and *Bifidobacterium*, also accompanied by a decrease in *Lactobacilli* [42] and their positive effects on the health of the host. Likewise, several authors have highlighted the variations between the number of facultative anaerobes in adults and the elderly [43, 44].

Many bacterial species are commensal flora in the intestine, and others are highly pathogenic such as *Helicobacter pylori*, *Salmonella enterica*, *Salmonella* Enteritidis, *Salmonella* Heidelberg, *Salmonella* Typhimurium, *Shigella dysenteriae*, *Clostridium difficile*, *Klebsiella* spp., *Enterobacter* spp., *Vibrio* spp., *Yersinia pestis*, *Proteus spp*., *Bacillus cereus, Campylobacter coli*, *Campylobacter jejuni*, and enterotoxigenic *Escherichia coli*, which cause gastrointestinal diseases with different pathogenesis according to age, gut health, chronic diseases, and immune diseases, among other triggers. Gut disturbances in the microbiota may cause dysbiosis and bacterial translocation, mediated by lipopolysaccharide binding to Toll-like receptor 4 (TLR4) and the transcription factor nuclear factor NFκB as an inflammatory response. These mechanisms origin damage in gut barrier integrity and immune system of this organ [29, 45–49] (**Table 1**).

Phytochemical compounds	Sources	Part used	Model experiment	Outcomes	References
Polyphenols					
Phenolic acids, stilbenoids, flavonols, dihydroflavonols, and anthocyanins	*Vitis vinifera*	Fruits	Humans	↑*Enterococcus* spp., *Prevotella* spp., *Bifidobacterium* spp., *B. uniformis*, *E. lento*, *B. coccoides*, *E. rectale*	[50]
Chlorogenic acid-polyphenols	Green coffee	Bean	High fat-fed mice	↑*Bacteroides*, *Bifidobacterium*, *Lactobacillus*, *Ruminococcaceae* ↓*Desulfovibrionaceae*, *Lachnospiraceae*, *Erysipelotrichaceae*	[51]
Phenolic compounds	*Allium sativum*	Whole plant	In vitro	↓*S. epidermidis*, *K. pneumoniae*	[52]
Tannins	*Moringa oleifera*	Leaves	Mice	↓ *Clostridium leptum*, ↑*Bacteroides*	[47–49, 53]
Anthocyanidins and flavonoids	*Punica granatum*	Fruits	Mice and high fat-fed mice	↑*Lactobacillus* spp., *Bifidobacterium* ↓*E. coli*, *Salmonella* spp.	[21, 22, 54–56]
Anthocyanidins	*Rubus fruticosus* and *Rubus occidentalis*	Fruits	In vitro	↓*H. pylori*, *S. epidermis*, *K. pneumoniae*, *S. epidermis*, *K. pneumoniae*, *E. coli*, *Salmonella* spp.	[57–59]
Anthocyanidins	*Antirrhinum majus*	Flowers	High fat-fed mice	↑*Bifidobacterium* spp., *Lactobacillus* spp.	[22, 25]
Syringe, p-coumaric, 4-hydroxybenzoic, and vanillic	*Larix laricina*	Needles	Mice	↑*Bifidobacterium*, *Enterococcus*, *Eggerthella lenta*	[60]
Catechins, flavan-3-ols, and monomeric flavan-3-olrich rich	Green tea	Leaves	Humans	↓*S. mutans*, *Shigella*, *V. cholerae*, *C. histolyticum*, *C. coccoides-E. rectale* ↑*Lactobacillus* spp.	[59, 61, 62]
Procyanidins, catechin and epicatechin	*Pyrus malus*	Fruits	Mice	↑*Bifidobacterium* spp.	[63]
Gallic acids	*Phyllanthus niruri* and *Moringa oleifera*	Leaves	Mice	↓*E. coli*, *P. aeruginosa*	[64, 65]
Coumarins					
Coumarins	*Anacardium occidentale*	Leaves	In vitro	↓*Staphylococcus aureus*	[66]
6′,7′-dihydroxy-bergamottin, officinalin, stenocarpin isobutyrate, officinalin isobutyrate, 8-methoxypeucedanin, and peucedanin	*Peucedanum luxurians*	Fruits	In vitro	↓*E. coli*, ↓*Salmonella* spp.	[67]

Phytochemical compounds	Sources	Part used	Model experiment	Outcomes	References
Coumarin-1,2,3-triazole conjugate and 3-heteroarylazo 4-hydroxy	*Synthesized*		In vitro	↓*E. faecalis, S. aureus, E. coli, B. subtilis, P. aeruginosa*	[49, 68, 69]
Triterpenes					
Terpineol	*Cinnamomum verum*	Whole plant	In vitro	↓*H. pylori*	[24]
Petalostemumol	*Dalea purpurea* and *Vitis vinifera*	Flowers	In vitro	↓*B. subtilis, S. aureus, Candida albicans*	[47, 70]
1α, 3β, 23-trihydroxyolean-12-in-29-oic acid	*Combretum imberbe*	Cortex	In vitro	↓*M. fortuitum, S. aureus*	[71]
23-hydroxyursolic acid, hederagenin, 3-O-α-L-arabinopyranosyl-echinocystic acid, 3-O-α-L-arabinopyranosyl-oleanolic acid, and 3-O-α-L-arabinopyranosyl-ursolic acid	*Cussonia bancoensis*	Stem bark	In vitro	↓*S. aureus, S. pyogenes, E. faecalis, S. Typhi, C. albicans*	[72]
Alkaloids					
4-methoxy-1-methyl-quinolin-2- (1H) -one	*Pleurothyrium cinereum, Esenbeckia alata* and *Raputia heptaphylla*	Leaves	In vitro	↓*E. faecalis, S. aureus, E. coli, S.* Typhimurium	
Sanguinarine, chelerythrine, protopine and allocryptopine and phenolics, gallic, protocatechuic, p-hydroxybenzoic, m-hydroxybenzoic, gentisic, p-coumaric, caffeic, ferulic, and sinapic acids	*Macleaya cordata*	Roots and leaves	In vitro	↓*S. aureus, E. coli, Salmonella* spp.	[73, 74]
Sanguinarine and dihydrosanguinarine	*Argemone mexicana*	Seeds and leaves	In vitro	↓*E. coli, P. aeruginosa*	[75]

Table 1.
Some phytochemical compounds that modulate gut microbiota.

Currently, many investigations focus on the search for therapeutic treatments through diet to modulate the intestinal microbiota, reducing inflammation in this organ, preventing chronic and degenerative diseases [22]. It has been shown that small concentrations of active ingredients from medicinal plants or other plant sources have microbiostatic and microbicidal activities against enteric pathogenic microbiota [76]. An increase of the competitive exclusion in the intestinal epithelium guarantees a greater metabolization of the phytochemical compounds by the bacteria and therefore benefits the biological response of the host [54, 77]. Although the mechanisms are not well, the phytochemical compounds can reduce the proliferation of pathogenic bacteria in the GIT, affect cell reproduction, mediate microbial metabolic processes, and regulate signal translation or genetic expression with phospholipoidal cell membranes, thus increasing the permeability and loss of cellular constituents, imbalance of the enzymes to the production of cellular energy and synthesis of organelle compounds, and destruction or inactivation of genetic material [45–48, 78].

3.1 Phenolic compounds

Scientific evidences show that within the phytochemical compounds, polyphenols are the most effective antimicrobials. In this sense, the phenolic compounds such as flavonols, flavones, and flavanones, and phenolic acids are poorly metabolizable by some gut microbiota. However, species such as *E. coli*, *Bifidobacterium* spp., *Lactobacillus* spp., *Bacteroides* spp., and *Eubacterium* spp. can catabolize these phenolic compounds and its fermentation products [49]. Also, colon bacteria metabolize the polyphenolic compounds into bioactive metabolites of low molecular weight easily absorbed by the organism [68].

The relationship between the most representative phylum of the intestine, *Firmicutes*/*Bacteroides*, is affected by phenolic compounds of vegetable origin [70]. A study in humans indicated that the consumption of polyphenols from *Vitis vinifera* rich in phenolic acids, stilbenoids, flavonols, dihydroflavonols, and anthocyanins significantly increased the number of *Enterococcus* spp., *Prevotella* spp., *Bifidobacterium* spp., *Bacteroides uniformis*, *Eggerthella lenta*, *Blautia coccoides*, and *Eubacterium rectale*, although the population of *Lactobacillus* spp. remained unchanged [50]. Also, in rats treated with chlorogenic acid-polyphenols (rich in green coffee bean), the concentration of beneficial bacteria such as *Bacteroides*, *Bifidobacterium*, and *Lactobacillus* spp. was significantly increased, while the composition of *Ruminococcaceae, Desulfovibrionaceae, Lachnospiraceae,* and *Erysipelotrichaceae* decreased with the experimental treatment [51]. Moreover, phenolic compounds extracted from *Allium sativum* juice decrease the growth of pathogenic bacteria such as *Staphylococcus epidermidis* and *Klebsiella pneumoniae* [52]. Likewise, in rats with diets rich in tannins (rich in *Moringa oleifera*), *Clostridium leptum* decreased, while *Bacteroides* increased significantly; apparently, this diet suppressed the bacterial cell proliferation by blocking proteolytic macerating enzymes and inactivating microbial adhesins and cell envelope transport proteins [47, 48, 53].

Several authors have reported the modulating effect of anthocyanidins on the colonic microbiota and some inflammatory markers [21, 22, 60]. Anthocyanidins have the ability to inhibit the growth of intestinal pathogenic bacteria; apparently an interaction exists between the phenolic compounds and the local microbiota specifically (mainly *Bifidobacterium*), which increases the anti-inflammatory activity [22, 54]. The species *Lactobacillus* spp. and *Bifidobacterium* spp. maintain the stability of the enzyme activity, especially the β-glucosidase; this enzyme acts as a catalyst in the metabolic reactions of anthocyanidins; thus this phytochemical in the treatment of gut-related diseases could stimulate the growth of these beneficial bacterial species [21]. Gastric and intestinal bacteria such as *Helicobacter pylori*, *Salmonella* spp., and *Bacillus cereus* were inhibited by the anthocyanidins extracted from *Rubus fruticosus* and *Rubus occidentalis* fruits; also, this secondary metabolite has a bacteriostatic effect in vitro against *Staphylococcus epidermis*, *Klebsiella pneumoniae*, and *Escherichia coli* [57–59]. Other results showed that expression of *Bifidobacterium* spp. and *Lactobacillus* spp. increased with the consumption of anthocyanidins (*Antirrhinum majus* flowers) rich in in maternal diets with high content of trans-fatty acids [22, 25]. Also, fecal concentration of *Bifidobacterium*, *Enterococcus*, and *Eggerthella lenta* is higher with the prolonged consumption of polyphenol-rich foods, as well as the urinary concentrations of the anthocyanin metabolites, such as syringe, p-coumaric, 4-hydroxybenzoic, and vanillic (*Larix laricina*), which have been positively correlated with bifidobacteria of the intestine [60].

Green tea has high concentrations of catechins, which belong to the group of flavonoids; these secondary metabolites have good effects against *Streptococcus mutans, Shigella*, and *Vibrio cholerae* proven in in vivo studies [79]. Other in vivo *and* in vitro studies with green tea extracts rich in flavan-3-ols and monomeric flavan-3-olrich rich found a modulation of the intestinal microbiota, which produced changes in beneficial bacteria such as *Lactobacillus* spp., inhibiting other groups such as *Clostridium* spp. [59, 61, 62]. On the other hand, catechins significantly inhibited the growth of *Clostridium histolyticum*, *E. coli*, and members of the *Clostridium coccoides*/*Eubacterium rectale* group, without affecting the growth of *Lactobacillus* spp. and *Bifidobacterium* spp. [62]. Also, the extract of *Punica granatum* (rich in flavonoids) increased *Bifidobacterium* spp. in the cecum of the mice with hypercholesterolemia, obesity, and inflammatory disorders induced with high-lipid diets [54]. Likewise, in other studies, the stilbenoid resveratrol, ellagitanins, and urolithin A in pomegranate (alcoholic extract) treatment are responsible for the competitive exclusion in the intestinal epithelium with a higher population of *Bifidobacterium* spp. and *Lactobacillus* spp. in mice [55, 56].

As an interesting fact, the increase of the *Clostridium coccoides*/*Eubacterium rectale* group is related to its capacity for metabolizing these flavonoid compounds. In this sense, in an experiment treatment with flavonoids such as procyanidins, catechin, and epicatechin (*Pyrus malus*), the authors found an increase in *Bifidobacterium* spp. in the colon and a decrease of the inflammation biomarkers such as prostaglandin E2, TNF-α, and leukotriene B4 [63]. Furthermore, the gallic acids (*Phyllanthus niruri* and *Moringa oleifera*) bind to bacterial dihydrofolate reductase (DHFR) enzymes, which reduces the bacterial population of *E. coli* through the inhibition of supercoiling activity and bonding of ATP and gyrase B, so that it binds to bacterial DNA, thereby modulating topoisomerase IV enzyme-mediated DNA cleavage and bacterial growth stasis [64, 65]. This means that several groups of polyphenols directly influence the intestinal bacterial population of the organism (**Table 1**).

3.2 Coumarins

According to the in vitro results, the family of coumarins and reducing carbohydrates abundant in the hexane, chloroform, and ethyl acetate extracts of the leaves of *Anacardium occidentale* are responsible for the antistaphylococcal activity [66]. Another in vitro study where they isolated 6′,7′-dihydroxybergamottin, officinalin, stenocarpin isobutyrate, officinalin isobutyrate, 8-methoxypeucedanin, and peucedanin from *Peucedanum luxurians* fruits found a positive response by reducing all challenged Gram-negative pathogenic bacteria, such as *E. coli* and *Salmonella* spp. [67]. At present, the synthesis of some phytochemical compounds from plants and fungi is one of the very novel forms of use. Many coumarins are synthesized in the lab and used as medicines for humans and animals. In this sense, coumarin-1,2,3-triazole conjugate and 3-heteroarylazo 4-hydroxy showed bactericidal action against *Enterococcus faecalis* [80] and *Staphylococcus aureus*, *Escherichia coli*, *Bacillus subtilis*, and *Pseudomonas aeruginosa* [69], respectively (**Table 1**).

3.3 Triterpenes

On the other hand, phytochemical compounds such as terpineol from *Cinnamomum verum* have antiulcer activity by reducing the infection by *Helicobacter pylori* in vitro [24]. The ethanol-soluble fraction of *Dalea purpurea* and *Vitis vinifera* has a terpenoid called petalostemumol, which showed excellent activity against *Bacillus subtilis*, *Staphylococcus aureus*, and *Candida albicans* and lesser activity against Gram-negative bacteria [47]. Likewise, triterpene 1α, 3β, and 23-trihydroxyolean-12-in-29-oic acid isolated *Combretum imberbe* which inhibited the in vitro growth of *Mycobacterium fortuitum* and *Staphylococcus aureus* [81]. In an in vitro study, triterpenes such as 23-hydroxyursolic acid, hederagenin, 3-O-α-L-arabinopyranosyl-echinocystic acid, 3-O-α-L-arabinopyranosyl-oleanolic acid, and 3-O-α-L-arabinopyranosyl-ursolic acid isolated from the stem bark of *Cussonia bancoensis* stopped the growth of *Staphylococcus aureus*, *Streptococcus pyogenes*, *Enterococcus faecalis*, *Salmonella typhi*, and *Candida albicans* [71] (**Table 1**).

3.4 Alkaloids

Other groups of phytochemicals with bactericidal or bacteriostatic importance are alkaloids. In an investigation, 4-methoxy-1-methyl-quinolin-2- (1H)—one obtained from three tropical plants such as *Pleurothyrium cinereum*, *Esenbeckia alata*, and *Raputia heptaphylla*—showed an effective reduction against *Enterococcus faecalis*, *Staphylococcus aureus*, *Escherichia coli*, and *Salmonella typhimurium* [72]. Isoquinoline alkaloids from the roots and leaves of *Macleaya cordata* such as sanguinarine, chelerythrine, their dihydro derivatives, protopine and allocryptopine and phenolics, and gallic, protocatechuic, p-hydroxybenzoic, m-hydroxybenzoic, gentisic, p-coumaric, caffeic, ferulic, and sinapic acids have antibacterial action against *Staphylococcus aureus*, *E. coli*, and *Salmonella* spp. [73, 74]. Also, the leaves and seeds of *Argemone mexicana*, another plant rich in isoquinolinic alkaloids such as sanguinarine and dihydrosanguinarine, have powerful bactericidal action in vitro against *E. coli* and *Pseudomonas aeruginosa* [75] (**Table 1**).

In general, the antimicrobial activities of several phytochemical compounds based on chemical studies, in vitro and in vivo, are known. However, due to the alimentary habit of a part of the world population, many of these medicinal compounds are not used, mainly as part of the diet, as aqueous extracts, or as alcoholic extracts, although other times they are used empirically, showing their beneficial effect. The daily use of phytochemicals in a controlled manner and according to scientific bases, both chemical and biological, could prevent or treat many ailments and diseases related to intestinal dysbiosis in humans.

4. Conclusions

This review has highlighted the role of the phytochemical compounds like modulators of gut microbiota. It was identified that alkaloids, steroids, phenols, flavonoids, glycosides, coumarins, quinones, tannins, and terpenoids are the main phytochemical compounds with biological activity. In addition, in vitro and in vivo experiments demonstrated that these beneficial chemical compounds can reduce the proliferation of pathogenic bacteria in the gastrointestinal tract through various biochemical and physiological processes that cause disturbances in the bacterial cell membrane, which causes competitive exclusion in the epithelial membrane by a greater expression of *Bifidobacterium* spp. and *Lactobacillus* spp., which reduce the appearance of dysbiosis, bacterial translocation, damage to the intestinal barrier, and gastrointestinal problems.

Conflict of interest

The authors declare no conflict of interest.

Author details

Yordan Martínez[1*] and Dairon Más[2]

1 Agricultural Sciences and Production Department, Zamorano Pan-American Agricultural School (Zamorano University), Honduras

2 Faculty of Natural Sciences, Laboratory of Animal Nutrition, Autonomous University of Queretaro, Queretaro, Mexico

*Address all correspondence to: ymartinez@zamorano.edu

References

[1] Newman DJ, Cragg GM, Snader KM. The influence of natural products upon drug discovery. Natural Product Reports. 2000;**17**:215-234. DOI: 10.1039/A902202C

[2] Fabricant DS, Farnsworth NR. The value of plants used in traditional medicine for drug discovery. Environmental Health Perspectives. 2001;**109**:69-75. DOI: 10.1289/ehp.01109s169

[3] Newman DJ, Cragg GM. Natural products as sources of new drugs over the last 25 years. Journal of Natural Products. 2007;**70**:461-477

[4] Shi Q, Li L, Huo C, Zhang M, Wang Y. Study on natural medicinal chemistry and new drug development. Chinese Traditional and Herbal Drugs. 2010;**41**:1583-1589

[5] Hosseinzadeh S, Jafarikukhdan A, Hosseini A, Armand R. The application of medicinal plants in traditional and modern medicine: A review of *Thymus vulgaris*. International Journal of Clinical Medicine. 2015;**6**:635-642. DOI: 10.4236/ijcm.2015.69084

[6] Madhumitha G, Elango G, Roopan SM. Biotechnological aspects of ZnO nanoparticles: Overview on synthesis and its applications. Applied Microbiology and Biotechnology. 2016;**100**:571-581. DOI: 10.1007/s00253-015-7108-x

[7] Ames BN, Shigenaga MK, Hagen TM. Oxidants, antioxidants, and the degenerative diseases of aging. Proceedings of the National Academy of Sciences. 1993;**90**:7915-7922. DOI: 10.1073/pnas.90.17.7915

[8] Boyer J, Liu RH. Apple phytochemicals and their health benefits. Nutrition Journal. 2004;**3**:5. DOI: 10.1186/1475-2891-3-5

[9] Akinpelu DA. Antimicrobial activity of *Anacardium occidentale* bark. Fitoterapia. 2001;**72**:286-287. DOI: 10.1016/S0367-326X(00)00310-5

[10] Velu G, Palanichamy V, Rajan AP. Phytochemical and pharmacological importance of plant secondary metabolites in modern medicine. In: Bioorganic Phase in Natural Food: An Overview. Berlin: Springer; 2018. pp. 135-156

[11] Anupama N, Madhumitha G, Rajesh KS. Role of dried fruits of *Carissa carandas* as anti-inflammatory agents and the analysis of phytochemical constituents by GC-MS. Biomed Research International. 2014;**2014**. DOI: 10.1155/2014/512369

[12] Nagulendran KR, Velavan S, Mahesh R, Hazeena BV. *In vitro* antioxidant activity and total polyphenolic content of *Cyperus rotundus* rhizomes. E-Journal of Chemistry. 2007;**4**:440-449. DOI: 10.1155/2007/903496

[13] Kamboj V. Herbal medicine. Current Science. 2000;**78**:35-39

[14] Sen S, Chakraborty R, De B. Joydeep Mazumder. Plants and phytochemicals for peptic ulcer: An overview. Pharmacognosy Reviews. 2009;**3**:270-279

[15] Albenberg LG, Wu GD. Diet and the intestinal microbiome: Associations, functions, and implications for health and disease. Gastroenterology. 2014;**146**:1564-1572. DOI: 10.1053/j.gastro.2014.01.058

[16] Fukuda S, Ohno H. Gut microbiome and metabolic diseases. Seminars In Immunopathology. 2014;**36**:103-114. DOI: 10.1007/s00281-013-0399-z

[17] Azad MAK, Sarker M, Li T, Yin J. Probiotic species in the modulation of

gut microbiota: An overview. Biomed Research International. 2018;**2018**:1-8. DOI: 10.1155/2018/9478630

[18] Mariat D, Firmesse O, Levenez F, Guimarães V, Sokol H, Doré J, et al. The Firmicutes/Bacteroidetes ratio of the human microbiota changes with age. BMC Microbiology. 2009;**9**:123. DOI: 10.1186/1471-2180-9-123

[19] Lay C, Sutren M, Rochet V, Saunier K, Dore J, Rigottier-Gois L. Design and validation of 16S rRNA probes to enumerate members of the *Clostridium leptum* subgroup in human faecal microbiota. Environmental Microbiology. 2005;**7**:933-946. DOI: 10.1111/j.1462-2920.2005.00763.x

[20] Cani PD, Neyrinck AM, Fava F, Knauf C, Burcelin RG, Tuohy KM, et al. Selective increases of bifidobacteria in gut microflora improve high-fat-diet-induced diabetes in mice through a mechanism associated with endotoxaemia. Diabetologia. 2007;**50**:2374-2383. DOI: 10.1007/s00125-007-0791-0

[21] Faria A, Fernandes I, Norberto S, Mateus N, Calhau C. Interplay between anthocyanins and gut microbiota. Journal of Agricultural and Food Chemistry. 2014;**62**:6898-6902. DOI: 10.1021/jf501808a

[22] Morais CA, de Rosso VV, Estadella D, Pisani LP. Anthocyanins as inflammatory modulators and the role of the gut microbiota. The Journal of Nutritional Biochemistry. 2016;**33**:1-7. DOI: 10.1016/j.jnutbio.2015.11.008

[23] Selma MV, Espín JC, Tomás-Barberán FA. Interaction between phenolics and gut microbiota: Role in human health. Journal of Agricultural and Food Chemistry. 2009;**57**:6485-6501. DOI: 10.1021/jf902107d

[24] Jakhetia V, Patel R, Khatri P, Pahuja N, Garg S, Pandey A, et al. Cinnamon: A pharmacological review. Journal of Advanced Scientific Research. 2010;**1**:19-23

[25] Morais CA, Oyama LM, de Moura CR, de Rosso VV, do Nascimento CO, Pisani LP. Polyphenols-rich fruit in maternal diet modulates inflammatory markers and the gut microbiota and improves colonic expression of ZO-1 in offspring. Food Research International. 2015;**77**:186-193. DOI: 10.1016/j.foodres.2015.06.043

[26] Buchanan B, Gruissem W, Jones R. Biochemistry and Molecular Biology of Plants. New Jersey, USA: John Wiley & Sons; 2015

[27] Stamp N. Out of the quagmire of plant defense hypotheses. The Quarterly Review of Biology. 2003;**78**:23-55. DOI: 10.1086/367580

[28] Kabera JN, Semana E, Mussa AR, He X. Plant secondary metabolites: Biosynthesis, classification, function and pharmacological properties. The Journal of Pharmacy and Pharmacology. 2014;**2**:377-392

[29] Kumar S, Pandey A. Free radicals: Health implications and their mitigation by herbals. British Journal of Medicine and Medical Research. 2015;**7**:438-457. DOI: 10.9734/bjmmr/2015/16284

[30] Yildirim A, Oktay M, Bilaloglu V. The antioxidant activity of the leaves of *Cydonia vulgaris*. Turkish Journal of Medical Sciences. 2001;**31**:23-27

[31] Dash DK, Yeligar VC, Nayak SS, Ghosh T, Rajalingam R, Sengupta P, et al. Evaluation of hepatoprotective and antioxidant activity of *Ichnocarpus frutescens* (Linn.) r.Br. On paracetamol-induced hepatotoxicity in rats. Tropical Journal of Pharmaceutical Research. 2011;**6**:755-765. DOI: 10.4314/tjpr.v6i3.14656

[32] Kagan VE, Kisin ER, Kawai K, Serinkan BF, Osipov AN, Serbinova EA,

et al. Toward mechanism-based antioxidant interventions: Lessons from natural antioxidants. Annals of the New York Academy of Sciences. 2002;**959**:188-198. DOI: 10.1111/j.1749-6632.2002.tb02093.x

[33] Madziga HA, Sanni S, Sandabe UK. Phytochemical and elemental analysis of *Acalypha wilkesiana* leaf. Journal of American Science. 2010;**6**:510-514

[34] Gritz EC, Bhandari V. The human neonatal gut microbiome: A brief review. Frontiers in Pediatrics. 2015;**3**:17. DOI: 10.3389/fped.2015.00017

[35] Lin L, Zhang J. Role of intestinal microbiota and metabolites on gut homeostasis and human diseases. BMC Immunology. 2017;**18**:2. DOI: 10.1186/s12865-016-0187-3

[36] Conlon MA, Bird AR. The impact of diet and lifestyle on gut microbiota and human health. Nutrients. 2015;**7**:17-44. DOI: 10.3390%2Fnu7010017

[37] Odamaki T, Kato K, Sugahara H, Hashikura N, Takahashi S, Xiao J, et al. Age-related changes in gut microbiota composition from newborn to centenarian: A cross-sectional study. BMC Microbiology. 2016;**16**:90. DOI: 10.1186/s12866-016-0708-5

[38] Ley R, Turnbaugh P, Klein S, Gordon J. Microbial ecology: Human gut microbes associated with obesity. Nature. 2006;**444**:1022. DOI: 10.1038/4441022a

[39] Quartieri A, Simone M, Gozzoli C, Popovic M, D'Auria G, Amaretti A, et al. Comparison of culture-dependent and independent approaches to characterize fecal bifidobacteria and lactobacilli. Anaerobe. 2016;**38**:130-137. DOI: 10.1016/j.anaerobe.2015.10.006

[40] Harmsen HJM, Raangs GC, He T, Degener JE, Welling GW. Extensive set of 16S rRNA-based probes for detection of bacteria in human feces. Applied and Environmental Microbiology. 2002;**68**:2982-2990. DOI: 10.1128/AEM.68.6.2982-2990.2002

[41] Palmer C, Bik EM, DiGiulio DB, Relman DA, Brown PO. Development of the human infant intestinal microbiota. PLoS Biology. 2007;**5**:e177. DOI: 10.1371/journal.pbio.0050177

[42] Milani C, Ticinesi A, Gerritsen J, Nouvenne A, Andrea Lugli G, Mancabelli L, et al. Gut microbiota composition and *Clostridium difficile* infection in hospitalized elderly individuals: A metagenomic study. Scientific Reports. 2016;**6**:25945. DOI: 10.1038/srep25945

[43] Backhed F, Ley R, Sonnenburg J, Peterson D, Gordon J. Host-bacterial mutualism in the human intestine. Science. 2005;**307**:1915-1920. DOI: 10.1126/science.1104816

[44] Arboleya S, Watkins C, Stanton C, Ross RP. Gut bifidobacteria populations in human health and aging. Frontiers in Microbiology. 2016;**7**:1204. DOI: 10.3389/fmicb.2016.01204

[45] Manson M. Cancer prevention–The potential for diet to modulate molecular signaling. Trends in Molecular Medicine. 2003;**9**:11-18. DOI: 10.1016/s1471-4914(02)00002-3

[46] Surh Y-J. Cancer chemoprevention with dietary phytochemicals. Nature Reviews. Cancer. 2003;**3**:768-780. DOI: 10.1038/nrc1189

[47] Omojate C, Enwa O, Jewo O, Eze O. Mechanisms of antimicrobial actions of phytochemicals against enteric pathogens–A review. Food Bioscience. 2017;**2**:85-91. DOI: 10.1016/j.fbio.2017.06.006

[48] Onyekaba T, Chinedu O, Fred AC. Phytochemical screening and investigations of antibacterial activities

of various fractions of the ethanol leaves extract of *Moringa oleifera* Lam (*Moringaceae*). International Journal of Pharmaceutical, Chemical & Biological Sciences. 2013;**3**:962-973

[49] Pacheco-Ordaz R, Wall-Medrano A, Goñi MG, Ramos-Clamont-Montfort G, Ayala-Zavala JF, González-Aguilar GA. Effect of phenolic compounds on the growth of selected probiotic and pathogenic bacteria. Letters in Applied Microbiology. 2018;**66**:25-31. DOI: 10.1111/lam.12814

[50] Queipo-Ortuño MI, Boto-Ordonez M, Murri M, Gomez-Zumaquero JM, Clemente-Postigo M, Estruch R, et al. Influence of red wine polyphenols and ethanol on the gut microbiota. The American Journal of Clinical Nutrition. 2012;**95**:1323-1334. DOI: 10.3945/ajcn.111.027847

[51] Wang Z, Lam K, Hu J, Ge S, Zhou A, Zheng B, et al. Chlorogenic acid alleviates obesity and modulates gut microbiota in high-fat-fed mice. Food Science & Nutrition. 2019;**7**: 579-588. DOI: 10.1002/fsn3.868

[52] Lee YL, Cesario T, Wang Y, Shanbrom E, Thrupp L. Antibacterial activity of vegetables and juices. Nutrition. 2003;**19**:994-996. DOI: 10.1016/j.nut.2003.08.003

[53] Moyo B, Masika PJ, Muchenje V. Antimicrobial activities of *Moringa oleifera* Lam leaf extracts. African Journal of Biotechnology. 2012;**11**: 2797-2802. DOI: 10.5897/AJB10.686

[54] Neyrinck AM, Van Hée VF, Bindels LB, De Backer F, Cani PD, Delzenne NM. Polyphenol-rich extract of pomegranate peel alleviates tissue inflammation and hypercholesterolaemia in high-fat diet-induced obese mice: Potential implication of the gut microbiota. The British Journal of Nutrition. 2013;**109**:802-809. DOI: 10.1017/S0007114512002206

[55] Larrosa M, Yañéz-Gascón MJ, Selma MV, González-Sarrías A, Toti S, Cerón JJ, et al. Effect of a low dose of dietary resveratrol on colon microbiota, inflammation and tissue damage in a DSS-induced colitis rat model. Journal of Agricultural and Food Chemistry. 2009;**57**:2211-2220. DOI: 10.1021/jf803638d

[56] Larrosa M, González-Sarrías A, Yáñez-gascón MJ, Selma MV, Azorín-Ortuño M, Toti S, et al. Anti-inflammatory properties of a pomegranate extract and its metabolite urolithin-a in a colitis rat model and the effect of colon inflammation on phenolic metabolism. The Journal of Nutritional Biochemistry. 2010;**21**:717-725. DOI: 10.1016/j.jnutbio.2009.04.012

[57] Puupponen-Pimia R, Nohynek L, Hartmann-Schmidlin S, Kahkonen M, Heinonen M, Maatta-Riihinen K, et al. Berry phenolics selectively inhibit the growth of intestinal pathogens. Journal of Applied Microbiology. 2005;**98**:991-1000. DOI: 10.1111/j.1365-2672.2005.02547.x

[58] Nohynek LJ, Alakomi H-L, Kähkönen MP, Heinonen M, Helander IM, Oksman-Caldentey KM, et al. Berry phenolics: Antimicrobial properties and mechanisms of action against severe human pathogens. Nutrition and Cancer. 2006;**54**:18-32. DOI: 10.1207/s15327914nc5401_4

[59] Molan AL, Liu Z, Kruger M. The ability of blackcurrant extracts to positively modulate key markers of gastrointestinal function in rats. World Journal of Microbiology and Biotechnology. 2010;**26**:1735-1743. DOI: 10.1007/s11274-010-0352-4

[60] Boto-Ordóñez M, Urpi-Sarda M, Queipo-Ortuño MI, Tulipani S, Tinahones FJ, Andres-Lacueva C. High levels of Bifidobacteria are associated with increased levels of anthocyanin microbial metaboli. Food & Function.

2014;**5**:1932-1938. DOI: 10.1039/c4fo00029c

[61] Tzounis X, Vulevic J, Kuhnle G, George T, Leonczak J, Gibson GR, et al. Flavanol monomer-induced changes to the human faecal microflora. The British Journal of Nutrition. 2008;**99**:782-792. DOI: 10.1017/S0007114507853384

[62] Tzounis X, Rodriguez-Mateos A, Vulevic J, Gibson GR, Kwik-Uribe C, Spencer JPE. Prebiotic evaluation of cocoa-derived flavanols in healthy humans by using a randomized, controlled, double-blind, crossover intervention study. The American Journal of Clinical Nutrition. 2011;**93**:62-72. DOI: 10.3945/ajcn.110.000075

[63] Espley RV, Butts CA, Laing WA, Martell S, Smith H, McGhie TK, et al. Dietary flavonoids from modified apple reduce inflammation markers and modulate gut microbiota in mice. The Journal of Nutrition. 2013;**144**:146-154. DOI: 10.3945/jn.113.182659

[64] Jayaraman P, Sakharkar MK, Lim CS, Tang TH, Sakharkar KR. Activity and interactions of antibiotic and phytochemical combinations against *Pseudomonas aeruginosa in vitro*. International Journal of Bological Sciences. 2010;**6**:556-568. DOI: 10.7150/ijbs.6.556

[65] Enwa FO, Omojate CG, Adonu C. A review on the phytochemical profile and the antibacterial susceptibility pattern of some clinical isolates to the ethanolic leaves extract of *Moringa oleifera* Lam (*Moringaceae*). International Journal of Advanced Research. 2013;**1**:226-238

[66] Martínez Aguilar Y, Rodríguez FS, Saavedra MA, Hermosilla Espinosa R, Yero OM. Secondary metabolites and *in vitro* antibacterial activity of extracts from *Anacardium occidentale* L.(cashew tree) leaves. Revista Cubana de Plantas Medicinales. 2012;**17**:320-329

[67] Widelski J, Luca SV, Skiba A, Chinou I, Marcourt L, Wolfender JL, et al. Isolation and antimicrobial activity of coumarin derivatives from fruits of *Peucedanum luxurians* Tamamsch. Molecules. 2018;**23**:1-12. DOI: 10.3390/molecules23051222

[68] Cardona F, Andrés-Lacuevac C, Tulipania S, Tinahonesb FJ, Queipo-Ortuño MI. Benefits of polyphenols on gut microbiota and implications in human health. The Journal of Nutritional Biochemistry. 2013;**24**:1415-1422. DOI: 10.1016/j.jnutbio.2013.05.001

[69] Sahoo J, Kumar Mekap S, Sudhir KP. Synthesis, spectral characterization of some new 3-heteroaryl azo 4-hydroxy coumarin derivatives and their antimicrobial evaluation. Journal of Taibah University for Science. 2015;**9**:187-195. DOI: 10.1016/j.jtusci.2014.08.001

[70] Hervert-Hernández D, Pintado C, Rotger R, Goñi I. Stimulatory role of grape pomace polyphenols on *Lactobacillus acidophilus* growth. International Journal of Food Microbiology. 2009;**136**:119-122. DOI: 10.1016/j.ijfoodmicro.2009.09.016

[71] Mireku EA, Mensah AY, Amponsah IK, Danquah CA, Anokwah D, Kwesi BM. Antimicrobial pentacyclic triterpenes and glycosides from the stem bark of *Cussonia bancoensis*. Natural Product Research. 2018;**10**:1-4. DOI: 10.1080/14786419.2018.1503262

[72] Suárez C, Enrique L, Barrera C, Andrés C, Coy Barrera E, Lozano MJ. Antibacterial activity of terpenes and alkaloids isolated from three Colombian plants. Revista Cubana de Farmacia. 2011;**45**:275-282

[73] Khin M, Jones AM, Cech NB, Caesar LK. Phytochemical analysis and antimicrobial efficacy of *Macleaya cordata* against extensively

drug-resistant *Staphylococcus aureus*. Natural Product Communications. 2019;**13**:1934578X1801301. DOI: 10.1177/1934578x1801301117

[74] Liu H, Wang J, Zhao J, Lu S, Wang J, Jiang W, et al. Isoquinoline alkaloids from *Macleaya cordata* active against plant microbial pathogens. Natural Product Communications. 2009;**4**:1557-1560. DOI: 10.1177/1934578x0900401120

[75] Singh A, Jain D, Upadhyay MK, Khandelwal N, Verma HN. Green synthesis of silver nanoparticles using *Argemone Mexicana* leaf extract and evaluation of their antimicrobial activities. Digest Journal of Nanomaterials and Biostructures. 2010;**5**:483-489

[76] Gouda S, Das G, Sen SK, Shin H-S, Patra JK. Endophytes: A treasure house of bioactive compounds of medicinal importance. Frontiers in Microbiology. 2016;**7**:1538. DOI: 10.3389/fmicb.2016.01538

[77] Abachi S, Lee S, Rupasinghe H. Molecular mechanisms of inhibition of *Streptococcus* species by phytochemicals. Molecules. 2016;**21**:215. DOI: 10.3390/molecules21020215

[78] Kris-Etherton PM, Hecker KD, Bonanome A, Coval SM, Binkoski AE, Hilpert KF, et al. Bioactive compounds in foods: Their role in the prevention of cardiovascular disease and cancer. The American Journal of Medicine. 2002;**113**(Suppl):71S-88S. DOI: 10.1016/s0002-9343(01)00995-0

[79] Di Lorenzo A, Nabavi SF, Sureda A, Moghaddam AH, Khanjani S, Arcidiaco P, et al. Antidepressive-like effects and antioxidant activity of green tea and GABA green tea in a mouse model of post-stroke depression. Molecular Nutrition & Food Research. 2016;**60**:566-579. DOI: 10.1002/mnfr.201500567

[80] López-Rojas P, Janeczko M, Kubiński K, Amesty Á, Masłyk M, Estévez-Braun A. Synthesis and antimicrobial activity of 4-substituted 1,2,3-triazole-coumarin derivatives. Molecules. 2018;**23**:1-18. DOI: 10.3390/molecules23010199

[81] Katerere DR, Gray AI, Nash RJ, Waigh RD. Antimicrobial activity of pentacyclic triterpenes isolated from African *Combretaceae*. Phytochemistry. 2003;**63**:81-88. DOI: 10.1055/s-0029-1234559

Chapter 3

Study Biochemistry of *Mentha longifolia* (L.) Huds.: A Review

Sadeq Sabeeh Kareem Al-Taie and Noor Falah Mahde Al-Kenane

Abstract

The *Mentha longifolia* were found to be a rich source of phytochemical compounds like piperitone, piperitone oxide, piperitenone, pulegone, d-limonene, menthone, carvone, menthol, β-caryophyllene, 1,8-cineole, 5,7,4-trihydroxy-6,2,3-trimethoxyflavone, carvone, limonene, tripal, and oxathiane. *Mentha longifolia* possess antioxidant effect that could be attributed to the presence of phytosterosls, unsaturated fatty acids, phenolic compounds, and specific volatile constituents and antimicrobial and interfere in the treatment of many diseases.

Keywords: biochemistry, *Mentha longifolia* (L.) Huds, essential oils, antioxidant activity

1. *Mentha* Linnaeus, Sp. Pl. 2: 576.1753

Mentha species belong to the family Lamiaceae (Labiatae) and are widely distributed in Asia, Africa, Europe, North America, and Australia [1].

Mentha is classified into 42 species including subspecies, varieties, cultivar, as well as several of hybrid species. There are five sections of *Mentha* genus: *Audibertia*, *Mentha*, *Eriodontes*, *Preslia*, and *Pulegium* [2]; this is classified according to genetic, cytological, and morphological features. The species of *Mentha grow in numerous and different environments.*

Mentha extracts have several traditional properties; it is used in foods and medicinal drugs. Literature search reported antioxidant, antimicrobial, antifungal, as well as effects against yeasts, and anti-inflammatory and sedative [3]. *Lamiaceae* species are carminative, treating of colds and flu, diuretic, respiratory tract problems, stomachache gastralgia, hemorrhoids and antispasmodic [4]. Phytochemical studies of *Mentha* showed the presence of phenolic compounds. Essential oil such as (limonene, carvone, β-caryophyllene, terpinen-4-ol, piperitenone, pulegone, 1,8-cineole, and menthol), terpenes, flavonoids, ascorbic acid [5].

2. Morphological character

Mentha longifolia (Linnaeus) Hudson (**Figure 1**).

Mentha longifolia is a creeping rhizomatous, perennial herb, opposite, two leaves per node. Sessile, it grows 30–100 cm tall, either hairless or hairy on the stems; the leaves are round, simple, lanceolate to oblong lanceolate, toothed, 1–3 cm long,

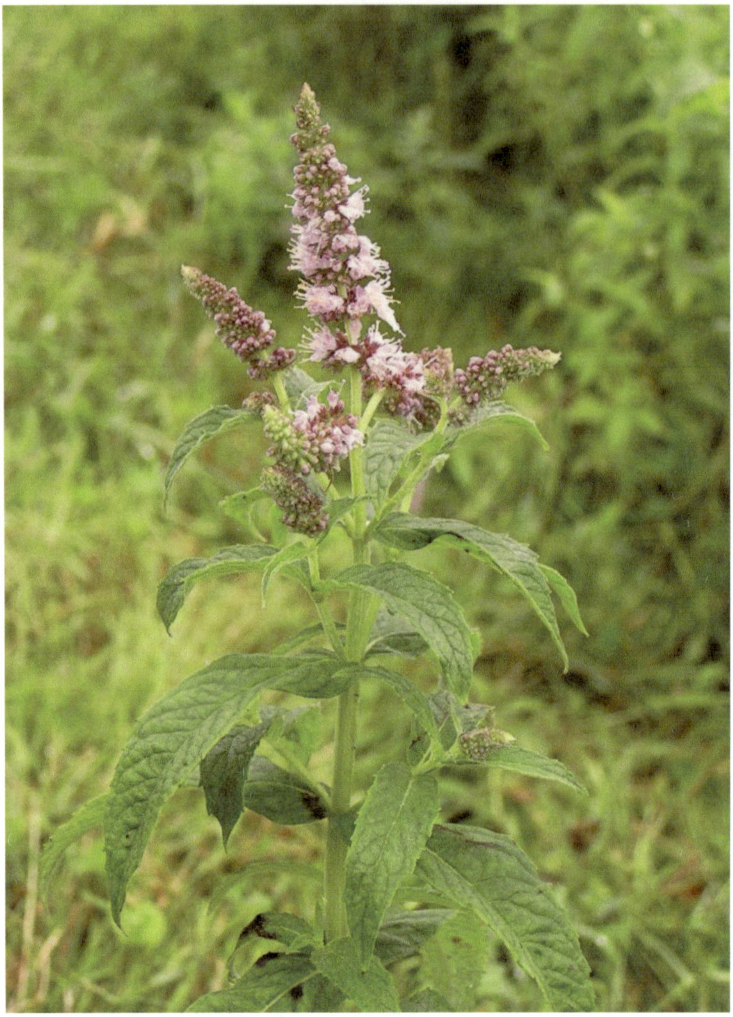

Figure 1.
Morphology of Mentha longifolia.

and 1.5–3 cm broad, smooth, or wrinkled with sharply serrate margin. The stem is erect, square-shaped, and light green to reddish green. Inflorescence, slender spikes produces pink, white, or lavender flowers in disrepute terminal spikes; bisexual, calyx short tubular, 1–2.5 mm, calyx short tubular, 1–2.5 mm, glabrous; corolla short tubular, 2–4 mm, with 5 lobes, white to pink, four stamens, subequal, pistil with a single style, exserted, the fruit is nutlets, dry, ovoid, and tuberculate, ovary smooth [6–9].

3. Phytochemistry of *Mentha longifolia* (Linnaeus) Hudson

The oils of *M. longifolia* are known to contain numerous monoterpenoids with piperitone oxide, piperitone, piperitenone, β-caryophyllene, d-limonene, carvone, menthone, pulegone1,8-cineole, and menthol as dominating compounds [5].

The phytochemical compounds of the essential oil of *M. longifolia* are studied by Moroccan [4] and reported that piperitenone oxide and piperitone oxide are the main compounds in the plant. In addition, five flavonoids and some non-volatile compounds are found such as *trans*-piperitone oxide, luteolin 7-*O*-glucoside and hesperidin, and piperitenone oxide luteolin. These compounds are used as antibacterial and against gastric problems and intraditional medicine [10, 11]. The essential oil of *M. longifolia* is represented by the oxygenated monoterpene group; this group includes 1,8-cineole, pulegone, piperitenone oxide [12, 13], and some other compound found in trace amounts such as sabinene, isomenthone, borneol, menthol, piperitenone, α-pinene, γ-terpineol, menthone, β-caryophyllene, isopulegone, and β-pinene.

Dzamic et al. [3] studied the *M. longifolia* in terms of its antioxidant and antifungal activity. They found that the constituents of the essential oils are about 35 chemical compounds. The highest compound was trans-dihydrocarvone (23.64%), and the lowest compound was cis-carveol and β-gurjunene (0.10%). As for minimal inhibitory (MIC) of *M. longifolia* essential oil (μl/ml), the values of some fungi were as follows:

1. 10 MIC in *Aspergillus flavus*, *A. ochraceus* and *Trichoderma viride*.

2. 5 MIC in *Alternaria alternate* and *Trichophyton mentagrophytes*.

3. 2.5 MIC in *Aspergillus niger*, *A. versicolor*, *Cladosporium fulvum*, *Fusarium tricinctum*, *F. sporotrichioides*, *Penicillium funiculosum*, *P. ochrochloron* and *Candida albicans*.

4. 1 MIC in *Cladosporium cladosporioides*.

The values of fungicidal concentrations (MFC) of *M. longifolia* essential oil (μl/ml) are as follows:

1. 10 MFC in *Alternaria alternate*, *Aspergillus niger*, *A. ochraceus*, *A. flavus*, *A, versicolor*, *Fusarium tricinctum*, *F. sporotrichioides*, *Penicillium funiculosum* and *Trichoderma viride*.

2. 5 MFC in *Trichophyton mentagrophytes* and *Candida albicans*.

3. 2.5 MFC in *Cladosporium cladosporioides*, *C. fulvum*, and *Penicillium ochrochloron*.

They also illustrate antioxidant activity of *M. longifolia* essential oil as shown in **Figure 2**.

The major components in the polish *M. longifolia* oil are limonene (5.8%), carvone (7.9%), 1,8-cineole (5.4%). and piperitone (4.8%) [14].

According to Khani and Asghari [15], the major volatile compounds were oxathiane (9.3%), tripal (14.3%), piperitenone (43.9%), piperitone oxide (5.9%), and d-limonene (4.3%) in *M. longifolia*.

The major volatile compounds of the Iranian *M. longifolia* oil were piperitone (43.9%), limonene (13.5%), and trans-piperitol (12.9%) [16]. Essential oil of *M. longifolia* showed some major component as; pulegone (21.90%), 1,8-cineole (11.58%), piperitone oxide (42.51%), and caryophyllene oxide (3.64%) [17].

The most abundant components in the essential oil of *M. longifolia* from Pakistani flora were borneol (5.96%), piperitenone (24.9%), piperitenone oxide

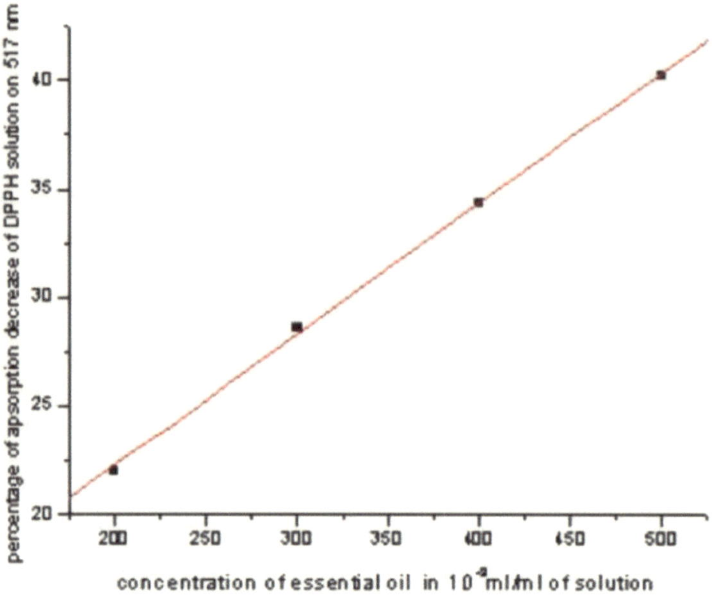

Figure 2.
Antioxidant activity of M. longifolia *essential oil [3].*

(28.3%), germacrene D (8.16%), and β-caryophyllene (5.94%), and the analyzed essential oil mainly consisted of oxygenated monoterpenes (67.24%) followed by sesquiterpene hydrocarbons (17.19%), monoterpene hydrocarbons (7.31%), and oxygenated sesquiterpenes (5.05%) [18].

Piperitone oxide and piperitenone oxide were the major components in the essential oil of *M. longifolia* from the middle Black Sea Region of Turkey [19].

In Egypt, a study prepared from *M. longifolia* aerial parts [20] found fatty acid content of the petroleum ether extracts of *M. longifolia* oil (the percentage of total fatty acids palimitic 1.63%, stearic 4.20%, linoleic 6.97%, and behenic 1.65%, total saturated fatty acids 7.488%, total unsaturated, fatty acids 6.97%), Gas liquid chromatography (GLC) analysis of unsaponifiable matter of M. longifolia oil (as percentage of total unsaponifiable matter) (hydrocarbon [higher alkanes], pentadecane 0.24%, hexadecane 0.03%, heptadecane 0.16%, octadecane 1.51%, nonadencane 15.94%, heneicosane 3.62%, docosane 10.548%, tetracosane 1.73%, hexacosane 0.576%, octacosane 4.09%, total hydrocarbon 38.47%, phytosterols [campesterol 3.37%, stigmasterol 1.87%, β-sitosterol 4.65%, total phytosterols 9.90%]) and chemical composition of hydrodistilled *M. longifolia* essential oil are α-pinene, sabinene, β-pinene, β-myrcene, limonene 1,8-cineole, linalool oxide, linalool, menthone, borneol, piperitone oxide, terpinehe-4-ol, α-terpineol, trans-carveol, thymole, piperitenone, piperitenone oxide, β-caryophyllene, humulene, D-germacrene, caryophyllene oxide, cedrol, α-cadinol, monoterpenes, oxygenated monoterpenes, sesquiterpene hydrocarbons, oxygenated sesquiterpene hydrocarbons.

M. longifolia essential oil belongs to oxygenated monoterpene group, which include pulegone, piperitenone oxide, and 1,8-cineole [12, 13] Beyond these, carvone, limonene, sabinene, α-pinene, isomenthone, borneol, menthol, menthone, piperitenone, dihydrocarvone eucalyptol, γ-terpineol, β-caryophyllene, isopulegone, cadinene, and β-pinene were also recorded as meaningful compounds from *M. longifolia* essential oil.

Component	Reference
Piperitone	[22]
Pulegone	[23, 24]
Cis-piperitone epoxide	[25]

Table 1.
The essential oils of M. longifolia *described in the literature.*

Identified chemical compounds	Reference
g, rosmarinic, salvianolic acid L	[26]
5-Hydroxy-6,7,3′,4′-tetramethoxyflavone	[3]

Table 2.
Major constituents of the phenolic composition and flavonoids of M. longifolia *described in the literature.*

The chemical compounds of some species of the genus Mentha are explained in [21], and the Mentha longifolia was among them, mentioning the essential oils as shown in **Table 1** and the phenolic compounds as shown in **Table 2** in the *M. longifolia*.

4. Phytochemistry in other species of the *Mentha* L.

As for the other species of the genus *Mentha*, it was rich in some chemical compounds, and it has a large antimicrobial role, including the *Mentha piperita* L. rich in caffeine, p-coumaric, ferulic, and rosmarinic acids that have an anti-*Staphylococcus aureus* and antiproliferative activity against two cancerous cell lines (MDA-MB-231), breast carcinoma cell line, and (A375) human melanoma cell line [27].

Patil et al. [28] reported that *Mentha piperita* is rich in chemical compounds such as diterpenes, tannins, flavonoids, cardiac glycosides, and stimulants, alkalis, phenols, coumarin, and saponins. These compounds have high activity as a microbial antibody.

Authors [29–31] also recorded menthofuran as an aromatic oil that ranges between 11 and 70.5% of the total content of the *Mentha aquatic*.

In *Mentha cervina* L. [32, 33], two compounds are mentioned; pulegone and isomenthone are the main components identified.

The *Mentha diemenica* essential oil in Australia was neomenthyl acetate, pulegone, and menthone, while the essential oil of the same species from Canada had significantly higher amounts of menthone, isomenthone and pulegone [34].

As mentioned by [13, 17], *Mentha spicata* L. essential oils are carvone and limonene.

Guedes *et al.* [35] found some chemical compounds in *Mentha arvensis* L. and *M. piperita* L. as shown in **Figure 3**.

The major component of essential oil in *M. arvensis* was menthol in the stem (78.16%), but it was (43.7%) in stolon (runner). Menthol is the major component of all the oils in *M. arvensis*, with the highest percentage in shoot stem oil (78.16%) and the lowest in stolon (runner) stem oil (43.7%). β-Caryophyllene oxide was the major component present in stem and leaf, while limonene, α-phellandrene, menthone, pulegone, and terpinolene are found in stolon [36].

Al-Okbi et al. [20] studied chemical content *Mentha citrate* shown in **Tables 3, 4** and **5**.

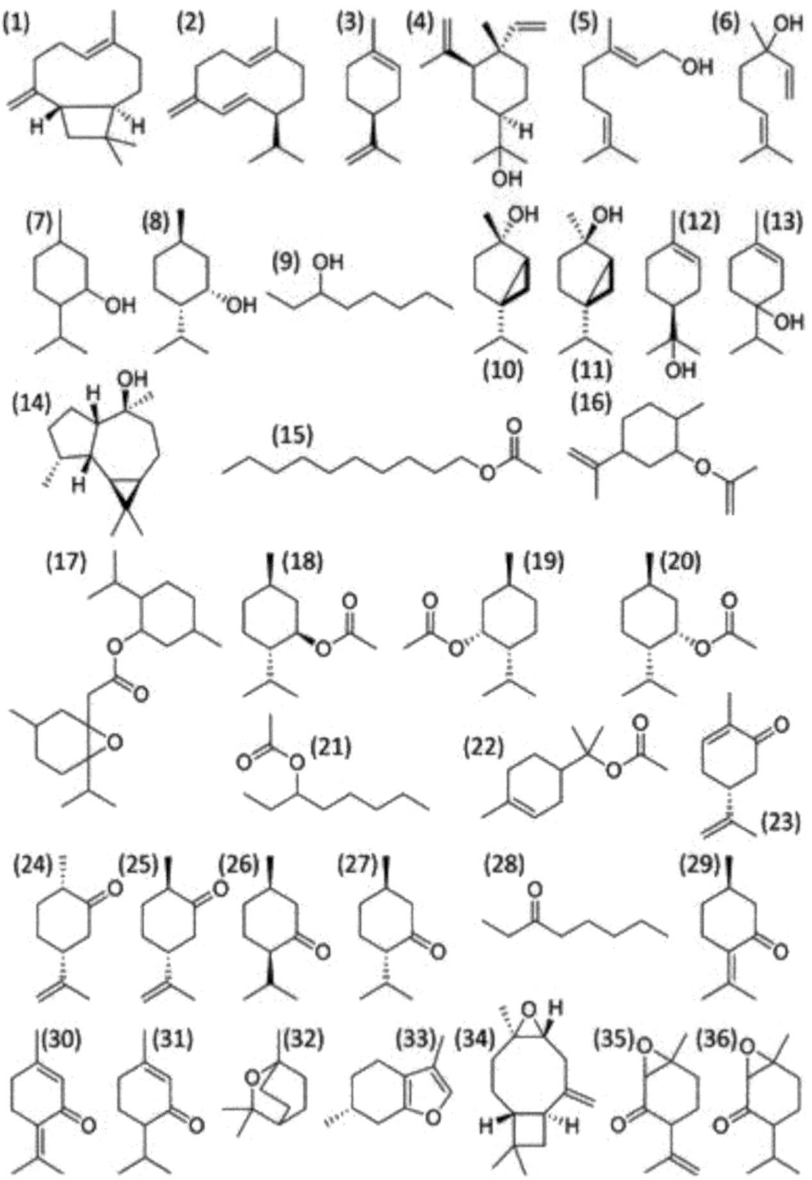

Figure 3.
Main components of Mentha *species essential oils: (1) β-caryophyllene, (2) germacrene D, (3) limonene, (4) elemol, (5) geraniol, (6) linalool, (7) menthol, (8) neomenthol, (9) 3-octanol, (10) cis-sabinene hydrate, (11) trans-sabinene hydrate, (12) α-terpineol, (13) terpinen-4-ol, (14) viridoflorol, (15) decyl acetate, (16) dihydrocarvyl acetate, (17) 1,2-epoxyneomenthyl acetate, (18) menthyl acetate, (19) neoisomenthyl acetate, (20) neomenthyl acetate, (21) 3-octyl acetate, (22) α-terpinyl acetate, (23) carvone, (24) cis-dihydrocarvone, (25) trans-dihydrocarvone, (26) isomenthone, (27) menthone, (28) 3-octanone, (29) pulegone, (30) piperitenone, (31) piperitone, (32) 1,8-cineole, (33) menthofuran, (34) caryophyllene oxide, (35) piperitenone oxide, and (36) piperitone oxide [35].*

Fatty acids	%
Palmitic	11.645
Stearic	8.437
Oleic	25.706
Linoleic	8.986
Behenic	3.777
Total saturated fatty acids	23.859
Total unsaturated fatty acids	34.692

Table 3.
Fatty acids' content of the petroleum ether extracts of Mentha citrata *oils (as percentage of total fatty acids) [20].*

Hydrocarbon and sterols	%
Hydrocarbon (higher alkanes)	
Hexadecane	0.005
Heptadecane	0.231
Octadecane	0.256
Nonadecane	0.527
Icosane	0.663
Heneicosane	0.142
Docosane	0.423
Tricosane	24.715
Tetracosane	1.816
Pentacosane	0.266
Hexacosane	4.217
Octacosane	6.792
Total hydrocarbon	40.053
Phytosterols	
Campesterol	4.284
Stigmasterol	0.341
β-Sitosterol	5.748
Total phytosterols	14.657

Table 4.
GLC analysis of unsaponifiable matter Mentha citrata *oils (as percentage of total unsaponifiable matter) [20].*

Components	%
Linalool	20.99
Isopulegol	0.17
Menthol	0.25
Phenyl ethylalcohol	1.32
α-Terpineol	2.89

Components	%
1,8-Cineole	2.82
β-Ocimene	1.01
α-Terpinolene	0.53

Table 5.
Some chemical compounds (%) isolated from M. citrata *[20].*

5. Antioxidant activity of *Mentha longifolia* (Linnaeus) Hudson

Iqbal et al. [18] showed dichloromethane and methanol extracts of *M. longifolia* to exhibit excellent antioxidant activity.

The antioxidant activity of methanol extract of *M. longifolia* is studied by Vladimir-Knezevid et al. [37], which they reported the presence of rosmarinic acid in the dried plants. Rosmarinic acid was found in the highest amount in most of *Mentha* species [38].

The antioxidant activity of *M. longifolia* methanol extract has been investigated in Saudi Arabia [39]. Phytochemical compounds and antioxidant activity of *M. longifolia* were studied by [36]. Essential oils have a high free radical scavenging capacity. So *M. longifolia* essential oil represented as a safe antiseptic addition in antioxidant and pharmaceuticals [40–43].

The antioxidant activity of *M. longifolia* in study [20] could be ascribed to the total phenolic contents that have been determined in methanol extract, along with the essential oil.

6. Traditional indications of *M. longifolia*

Have been used as [22, 25]:

1. Antimicrobial, anti-catarrhal, antispasmodic carminative, and antirheumatic

2. Antiemetic, sedative, diuretic, and aphrodisiac

3. Insect repellent and deworming

4. Treatment of headaches

5. Blood purifier

6. Digestive disorders, jaundice and gallstone

7. Dyspnea, common cold, asthma, and cough wound healing

8. And other uses

7. Conclusion

This review discusses the chemical constituent of *Mentha longifolia* and its antioxidant and antimicrobial effect and its role in alternative medicine in various regions of the world.

Essential oils and other chemical compounds in plant are natural products, which have been used for several applications in pharmaceutical, cosmetic, agricultural, and bioactivity example stems, leaves, and flowers.

Mentha genus encompasses several species used at medical, industrial, and nutritional levels. Most species contain essential oils and phenolic compound such as *M. longifolia, M. piperita, M. aquatic, M. cervina, M. diemenica, M. spicata*, and *M. arvensis* rich in essential oils and other compounds show activities of antioxidant and antimicrobial, and their essential oils and their derived extracts used as natural food preservatives.

Author details

Sadeq Sabeeh Kareem Al-Taie[1*] and Noor Falah Mahde Al-Kenane[2]

1 Department of Biology, College of Science, University of Misan, Iraq

2 Animal Production Department, College of Agriculture, University of Misan, Iraq

*Address all correspondence to: sadeq_altaie@yahoo.com; sas_altti@uomisan.edu.iq

References

[1] Krzyzanowska J, Janda B, Pecio L, Stochmal A, Oleszek W, Czubacka A. Determination of polyphenols in *Mentha longifolia* and *M. piperita* field-grown and in vitro plant samples using UPLC-TQ-MS. Journal of AOAC International. 2011;**94**(1):43-50

[2] Shekarchi M, Hajimehdipoor H, Saeidnia S, Gohari AR, Hamedani MP. Comparative study of rosmarinic acid content in some plants of Labiatae family. Pharmacognosy Magazine. 2012;**8**(29):37-41

[3] Dzamic AM, Marina DS, Mihailo SR, Miroslav N, Slavica G, Vele T, et al. Antifungal and antioxidant activity of *Mentha longifolia* (L.) Hudson (Lamiaceae) essential oil. Botanica Serbica. 2010;**34**(1):57-61

[4] Ertas A, Goren AC, Hasimi N, Tolan V, Kolak U. Evaluation of antioxidant, cholinesterase inhibitory and antimicrobial properties of *Mentha longifolia* subsp. noeana and its secondary metabolites. Records of Natural Products. 2015;**9**(1):105-115

[5] Oinonen PP, Jokela JK, Hatakka AI, Vuorela PM. Linarin, a selective acetylcholinesterase inhibitor from *Mentha arvensis*. Fitoterapia. 2006;**77**:429-434

[6] Al-Musawi AH. Plant Taxonomy. 1st ed. College of Science, University of Baghdad (in Arabic); 1987

[7] Bo He Shu. Mentha Flora of China. 1994;**17**:236-239

[8] Davis PH. Flora of Turkey and the East Aegen Island. Edinburgh University Press; 1967

[9] Gulluce M, Sahin F, Sokmen M, Ozer H, Daferera D, Sokmen A, et al. Antimicrobial and antioxidant properties of the essential oils and methanol extract from *Mentha longifolia* L. ssp. *longifolia*. Food Chemistry. 2007;**103**:1449-1456

[10] Banthorpe DV, Duprey RJH, Hassan M, Janes JF, Modawi BM. Chemistry of the Sudanese flora. Part II. Essential oil of *Mentha longifolia*. Egyptian Journal of Chemistry. 1980;**23**:63

[11] Patil SR, Patil RS, Godghate AG. *Mentha piperita* Linn: Phytochemical, antibacterial and dipterian adulticidal approach. International Journal of Pharmacy and Pharmaceutical Sciences. 2016;**8**(3):352-355

[12] Mikaili P, Mojaverrostami S, Moloudizargar IM, Aghajanshakeri S. Pharmacological and therapeutic effects of *Mentha longifolia* L. and its main constituent, menthol. Ancient Science of Life. 2013;**33**:129-136

[13] Mokaberinejad R, Zafarghandi N, Bioos S, Dabaghian HF, Naseri M, Kamalinejad M, et al. *Mentha longifolia* syrup in secondary amenorrhea: A double-blind, placebo-controlled, randomized trials. DARU Journal of Pharmaceutical Sciences. 2012;**20**:97

[14] Bertoli A, Leonardi M, Kryzyzanowska J, Oleszek W, Pistelli L. *Mentha longifolia in vitro* cultures as safe source of flavouring ingredients. Acta Biochemica Polonica. 2011;**58**(4):581-587

[15] Iqbal T, Hussain AI, Chatha SAS, Naqvi SAR, Bokhari TH. Antioxidant activity and volatile and phenolic profiles of essential oil and different extracts of Wild Mint (*Mentha longifolia*) from the Pakistani Flora. Journal of Analytical Methods in Chemistry. 2013. Article ID: 536490

[16] Rasooli I, Rezaei MB. Bioactivity and chemical properties of essential

oils from *Zataria multiflora* Boiss and *Mentha longifolia* (L.) Huds. Journal of Essential Oil Research. 2002;**14**(2)

[17] Mkaddem M, Bouajila J, Ennajar M, Lebrihi A, Mathieu F, Romdhane M. Chemical composition and antimicrobial and antioxidant activities of *Mentha* (*longifolia* L. and *viridis*) essential oils. Journal of Food Science. 2009;**74**:358-363

[18] Hajlaoui H, Trabelsi N, Noumi E, Snoussi M, Fallah H, Ksouri R, et al. Biological activities of the essential oils and methanol extract of tow cultivated mint species (*Mentha longifolia* and *Mentha pulegium*) used in the Tunisian folkloric medicine. World Journal of Microbiology and Biotechnology. 2009;**25**:2227

[19] Aksit H, Demirtas I, Telci I, Tarimcilar G. Chemical diversity in essential oil composition of *Mentha longifolia* (L.) Hudson subsp. typhoides (Briq.) Harley var. typhoides from Turkey. Journal of Essential Oil Research. 2013;**25**(5):430-437

[20] Al-Okbi SY, Hoda HM, Doha AM. Phytochemical constituents, antioxidant and anticancer activity of *Mentha citrata* and *Mentha longifolia*. Research Journal of Pharmaceutical, Biological and Chemical Sciences. 2015;**6**(1):739-751

[21] Brahmi F, Khodir M, Mohamed C, Duez Pierre D. Chemical Composition and Biological Activities of *Mentha* Species. Open Access Peer-Reviewed Chapter. 2017

[22] Mamadalieva NZ, Akramov DK, Ovidi E, Tiezzi A, Nahar L, Azimova SS, et al. Aromatic medicinal plants of the Lamiaceae family from Uzbekistan: Ethnopharmacology, essential oils composition and biological activities. Medicine. 2017;**4**:8

[23] Diop SM, Gueye MT, Ndiaye I, Ndiaye EB, Diop MB, Heuskin S, et al. Chemical composition of essential oils and floral waters of *Mentha longifolia* (L.) Huds. from Senegal. American Journal of Essential Oils and Natural Products. 2016;**4**(1):46-49

[24] Harley RM. Mentha. In: Tutin TG, Heywood VH, Burges NA, Moor DM, Valentine DH, Walters SM, Webb DA, editors. Flora Europaea III. Cambridge, UK: Cambridge University Press; 1972. pp. 183-186

[25] Guedes JP, Costa Medeiros JA, de Silva RSS, De Sousa JMB, Da Conceição ML, De Souza EL. The efficacy of *Mentha arvensis* L. and *M. piperita* L. essential oils in reducing pathogenic bacteria and maintaining quality characteristics in cashew, guava, mango, and pineapple juices. International Journal of Food Microbiology. 2016;**238**:183-192

[26] Khani A, Asghari J. Insecticide activity of essential oils of *Mentha longifolia*, *Pulicaria gnaphalodes* and *Achillea wilhelmsii* against two stored product pests, the flour beetle, *Tribolium castaneum*, and the cowpea weevil, *Callosobruchus maculates*. Journal of Insect Science. 2010;**12**:73

[27] Alexa E, Danciu C, Radulov I, Obistioiu D, Sumalan R, Morar A, et al. Phytochemical screening and biological activity of *Mentha×piperita* L. and *Lavandula angustifolia* Mill. extracts. Analytical Cellular Pathology. 2018;**2018**:7. Article ID: 2678924

[28] Oyedeji OA, Afolayan AJ. Chemical composition and antibacterial activity of the essential oil isolated from South African *Mentha longifolia* (L.) L. subsp. *capensis* (Thunb.) Briq. Journal of Essential Oil Research. 2006;**18**:57-59

[29] Başer K, Kurkcuoglu M, Demirci B, Ozek T, Tarımcılar G. Essential oils of *Mentha* species from marmara region of Turkey. Journal of Essential Oil Research. 2012;**24**:265-272

[30] Boz I, Zamfirache MM, Burzo I. Chemical composition of essential oils from *Mentha aquatica* L. at different moments of the ontogenetic cycle. Journal of Medicinal Plants Research. 2013;**7**:470-473

[31] Do Ngoc Dai TDT, Emmanuel EE, Oladimeji O, Abdulkabir IAO. Study on essential oil of *Mentha aquatica* L. from Vietnam. American Journal of Essential Oils and Natural Products. 2015:212-216

[32] Ghoulami S, Abdelkader I, Fkih-Tetouani IS. Phytochemical study of *Mentha longifolia* of Morocco. Fitoterapia. 2001;**72**:596-598

[33] Quezel P, Santa S. Nouvelle flore de l'Algerie et des regions desertiques meridionales. II. Ed. du C.N.R.S.; 1963

[34] Brophy JJ, Goldsack RJ, Lawrence BM, Forster PI. Essential oil of *Mentha diemenica* (Lamiaceae). Journal of Essential Oil Research. 1996;**8**:179-181

[35] Gonçalves M, Vicente A, Cavaleiro C, Salgueiro L. Composition and antifungal activity of the essential oil of *Mentha cervina* from Portugal. Natural Product Research. 2007;**21**:867-871

[36] Niksic H, Kovac-Besovis E, Makarevic E, Duric K. Chemical composition, antimicrobial and antioxidant properties of *Mentha longifolia* (L.) Huds. essential oil. Journal of Health Sciences. 2012;**2**(3):192-200

[37] Tucker AO. Mentha: Economic uses. In: Lawrence BM, editor. The Genus Mentha. Boca Raton, FL, USA: CRC Press, Taylor & Francis Group; 2007. pp. 519-522

[38] Salehi B, Zorica S, Jelena M, Farukh S, Hubert A, Dorota K, et al. Plants of Genus *Mentha*: From farm to food factory. Plants Review. 2018;**7**(3):70-95

[39] Al-Ali KH, El-Beshbishy HA, El-Badry AA, Alkhalaf M. Cytotoxic activity of methanolic extract of *Mentha longifolia* and *Ocimum basilicum* against human breast cancer. Pakistan Journal of Biological Sciences. 2013;**16**(23):1744-1750

[40] Chowdhury JU, Nandi NC, Uddin M, Rahman M. Chemical constituents of essential oils from two types of spearmint (*Mentha spicata* L. and *M. cardiaca* L.) introduced in Bangladesh. Bangladesh Journal of Scientific and Industrial Research. 2007;**42**:79-82

[41] Dwivedy AK, Prakash B, Chanotiya CS, Bisht D, Dubey NK. Chemically characterized *Mentha cardiaca* L. essential oil as plant based preservative based on efficacy against biodeteriorating fungi of dry fruits, aflatoxin secretion, lipid peroxidation and safety profile assessment. Food and Chemical Toxicology. 2017;**106**:175-184

[42] Rodrigues L, Monteiro P, Póvoa O, Teixeira G, Moldão M, Figueiredo AC, et al. Morphology of secretory structures and essential oil composition in *Mentha cervina* L. from Portugal. Flavour Fragrance Journal. 2008;**23**:340-347

[43] Vladimir-Knezevid S, Blazekovid B, Kindl M, Vladid J, Lower-Nedza AD, Brantner AB. Acetylcholinesterase inhibitory, antioxidant and phytochemical properties of selected medicinal plants of the Lamiaceae family. Molecules. 2014;**19**:767-782

Chapter 4

Rhus coriaria (Sumac): A Magical Spice

Thukaa Zuhair Abdul-Jalil

Abstract

Rhus coriaria L. (Sumac) has been used as folk medicine since ancient times. Rhus genus has over 91 of accepted species names in the Anacardiaceae family, *Rhus coriaria* L. is the only species in Iraq that growth wildly and/or cultivated near the villages in the north of Iraq. It has a characteristic taste and morphological features, making it to be considered as one of the popular flavoring spice, drink, appetizer, and as acidulant in food recipes, in addition to its role as plant medicine. A scrutiny of literature revealed some notable pharmacological activities of the plant such as antioxidant, anti-ischemic, antimicrobial as well as hypoglycemic and hypolipidimic effects. This chapter attempts to comprise the published obtainable literatures on *Rhus coriaria* with respect to its pharmacognostic characters, ethanobotanical/traditional uses, chemical constituents and summary of its various pharmacological activities, clinical effects, functional food industries and dentistry.

Keywords: spices, *Rhus coriaria* L., traditional uses, chemical constituents, pharmacological activities, functional food industries

1. Introduction

The old say of "Let food be the medicine and medicine be the food," by Hippocrates over 2500 years ago is gold shinning of the era today, as food interesting personals (scientist, suppliers and consumers) get the point of benefits for specific foods which have ingredients aiding some body functions as do improve health well-being [1].

From historic ages the discovery of spices had main role in the lifestyle of people in the old world. Spices are used for flavoring and coloring as do for food preserving for many millenniums as do its possession of medicinal properties using them in the traditional medicine has been authenticated since ancient times [2]. Today, spices are upgrading not only for their culinary properties but also for their potential health properties, as the advancement in its uses and acknowledgement of their chemistry, active constituent's pharmacodynamics/kinetics and health benefits affecting their investigation thoroughly in last decades. Hundreds of the adjuncts for food had been identified and authenticated by pioneering their health effects by observing research's on animals and human trials for them [3].

Sumac is the widespread name of the Rhus genus, which composes 91 of accepted species names in the Anacardiaceae family, represented in Iraq by one species namely *Rhus coriaria* L. which grow wildly and/or cultivated near the villages in the north of Iraq [4]. The "Sumac" name is derived from "summāq" that refer to "dark red" in Arabian and henceforth applied for the spice product of *Rhus coriaria* which had been utilized in spice mixtures in the Asian traditional medicines since ancient times [5].

Sumac had been implicated as a condiment spice in both pure and combination form spices. In Iraq, traditionally used with famous Iraqi meat dishes like Kabab, grilled meat as well as over salads served with them [4]. The *Rhus coriaria* extracts researched properties up-to-date revealed a promising potential furnishing renewable bio-products with desirable bioactivities like antimicrobial, antifungal, antiviral, antimalarial, antimutagenic, antioxidant, antimigratory, anti-ischemic, hypoglycemic and hypolipidimic affections [6].

In this chapter, a workup had been done to encompass the published literatures dealing with *Rhus coriaria* focusing on its pharmacognostic characters, ethanobotanical/traditional uses, and chemical constituents with summarizing its health promoting activities, clinical effects, applied functional foods industries and dentistry.

2. Taxonomical classification

Kingdom: Plantae
Sub kingdom: Tracheobionta
Super division: Spermatophyta
Division: Magnoliophyta
Subclass: Rosidae
Order: Sapindales
Family: Anacardiaceae
Genus: Rhus
Species: *Rhus coriaria* Linn
Vernacular Names.

Sumac (fruit of *Rhus coriaria* Linn) is known by different names worldwide including:

Persian: Samaka, Samak, Sumaq
Hindi: Tatrak, Tatri
Arabic: Timtima, Tamtam, Sumak, Sumac
Urdu: Sumaq
English: Sumach, Sumak
Bengali: Sumok
Kashmiri: Samak [7].

3. Habitat and distribution

The plant is wildly and/or cultivated in temperate and tropical regions of the continents with ability to grow on river sides lands. *Rhus coriaria* have superficial pervasion roots that can decrease ground drift and can be implanted on poorly eroded soils. Sumac commercially grown type is *Rhus coriaria* in the Mediterranean and Middle East, had been cultivated for several centuries to produce a material of high quality for tanning, also wildly in the territories from the Canary Island to the Mediterranean beaches to Afghanistan as it is municipal to the Mediterranean and the Southeastern territory of Turkey [6, 8]. While in Iraq, it's mostly found in North, North East and North West of it in areas of an altitude more than 540 m above sea level. Most researches with sumac interest say that *Rhus coriaria* grow in mountain environments especially in Amadia, Sinjar, Rawandowz and Sulimania which are the most prevalent territories [4].

4. Botanical description

Rhus coriaria is a small tree (shrub) with a height of up to 10 m (**Figure 1a**), its leaves are spirally coordinated with pinnately compound, with trifoliate or simple leaves in some species (**Figure 1b**). Its flowers are in spikes or dense panicles of 5–30 cm long, usually very small, with different colors (greenish, creamy white or red), with five petals (**Figure 1c**). It has small dark brown, laterally compressed

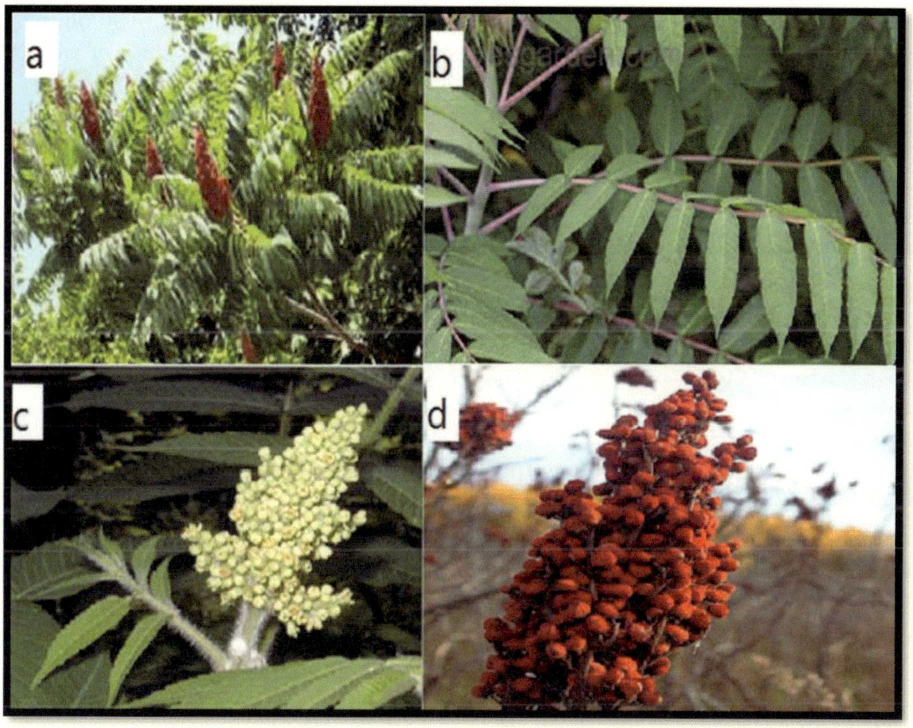

Figure 1.
Photo of Rhus coriaria *different parts: (a) shrub; (b) leaves; (c) flowers and (d) fruits.*

hard and hairy drupe fruits of diameters (length 3.5–4.0 cm and width 2–2.5 cm) permanent calyx, configuring dense panicles of reddish drupes clusters (**Figure 1d**) called sumac. The dried clusters are usually ground to produce a tangy purple spice. The seeds are little hard, brown colored with diameters (length 0.3–0.5 cm and width 0.2–o.3 cm) and good odor spicy [5, 6, 9].

5. Ethanobotanical and traditional uses

Rhus coriaria is a natural traditional medication fountain in many world dietary cultures, it is seasoning and flavoring used agent as a main pole in the municipal traditional remedies all over the globe. *Rhus coriaria* is a temptating ancient cooking in and over foods. About 2000 years ago, the "De Materia Medica" ("Of Medical Matters") a voluminous Greek physician book by the Pedanius Dioscorides (40–90 A.D.) had between its folds plentiful healthy merits of Sumac, mainly described as an anti-flatulent, stomach tonic and a diuretic. *Rhus coriaria* has been used commonly in the remedy of ulcer, anal piles, hepatic disease, diarrhea, animal bites, and pain management. Also for treatment of pharynx cold inflammations and seizing hemorrhage like hematemesis, hemoptysis, hemorrhoids and dysentery, it had been prescribed for ocular diseases like conjunctivitis, leucorrhea and ophthalmia. Conventional medicinal practice use *Rhus coriaria* for cholesterol reduction and in gynecology as an abortifacient. Others also report its use in improving wound healing and as an antimicrobial. Different parts of *Rhus coriaria* had been used in different recipes in indigenous herbal medicine.

Rhus coriaria bark powder is an effective teeth cleaning agent, while its infusion is useful in viral eye infections treatment while the water bruised is applied on the forehead for the first-aid treatment of epistaxis. Powdered fruits are sparsed on boiled eggs and eaten for the treatment of diarrhea. A fruits decoction is set and given orally (150 cc) trice daily for the treatment of hepatic diseases, urinary system disorders and diarrhea till improvement occurs [5, 6, 9–11].

6. Chemical constituents of *Rhus coriaria*

Until now, over 200 compounds have been identified from the *Rhus coriaria* and most of them are physiologically active. These chemical constituents can be assigned to various classes of the hydrolysable tannins, phenolic acids, conjugated phenolic acids, anthocyanins, flavonoids, organic acids, coumarins, xanthones, terpenoids, steroids, essential oils, and other groups of constituents have been reported. Summarization of the proportion of different chemical constituents of *Rhus coriaria* is shown in **Figure 2** [12].

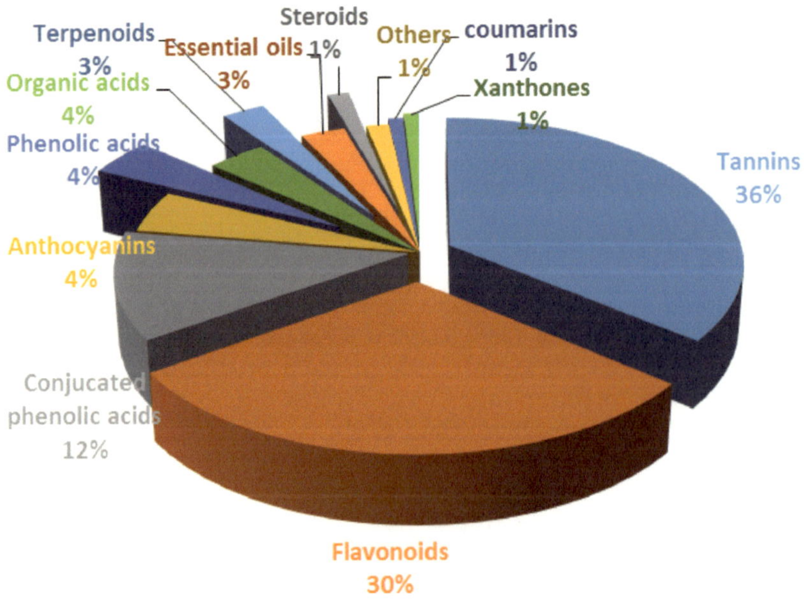

Figure 2.
Different subtype's comparison of the 200 constituents reported from Rhus coriaria.

Several phytochemical investigations for the constituents of *Rhus coriaria* and different part of the plant had been studied. Fruits are the most well researched part in which most of the chemical constituents had been detected. *Rhus coriaria* parts like leaves and seeds were also documented to hold a number of phyto-constituents as shown in **Table 1**.

Classes	Some important phyto-constituents	Parts of plant
Hydrolysable tannins	Gallic acid, methyl gallate, digallic acid, tri-gallic acid, ellagic acid, galloylhexose, O-galloylnorbergenin, O-galloyl arbutin.	Fruits ,leaves, seed
Phenolic acids	Protocatechuic acid syringic acid coumaryl-hexoside, caffeoylquinic acid *p*-benzoic acid, vanilic acid.	Fruits
Conjugated phenolic acids	Galloyl-hexose-malic acid, digalloyl-hexose malic acid, kaempferol hexose-malic acid, Myricetin hexose malic acid, quercetin-hexose malic acid. Isorhamnetin hexose-malic acid	Fruits
Anthocyanins	Cyaniding, peonidin, pelargonidin, petunidin, coumarates, delphinidin, Myrtillin and crysanthemin.	Fruits
Flavonoids	Quercetin, Isoquercitrin, quercitrin, Rutin, Kampferol, Myricetin ,apigenin Isorhamnetin, isovitexin, rhamnetin, ampelopsin	Leaves, fruits, seed
	Isoflavonoids: Glycitein-O-glucoside, oxoglycyrrhetinic acid.	Fruits
	Flavonoid dimers Amenthoflavone,agathisflavone ,hinokiflavone and sumaflavone	Fruits, leaves
Organic acids	Malic acid, Citric acid, Tartaric acid, Linoleic acid, Oleic acid, Linolenic acid, Palmitic acid and Stearic acid	Fruits ,Seed
Coumarins	Umbelliferon	Fruits
xanthones	2, 3-dihydroxy-7-methyl xanthone, 2, 3, 6-trihydroxy-7-hydroxymethylene xanthone-1-carboxylic acid and 2- methoxy- 4- hydroxy-7-methyl-3-*O*-beta-D-glucopyranosyl xanthone-1, 8-dicarboxylic Acid.	Seeds
Terpenoids	betunolic acid, A-tocopherol ,tocopherol mannoside, farnesylacetate, pentadecanal, hexadecanal, , deacetylforskolin, Oxoglyoyrrhotinic acid	Leaves, Fruits
Steroids	ß- sitosterol	Fruits, seed
Essential oils	(E)-Caryophyllene ,n-nonanal , cembrene, α-pinene (2E,4E)-decadienal nonanoic acid, (2E)-decenal, p-anisaldehyde, (Z)-2-decenal and caryophyllene oxide	Fruits
Others Butein	chalconoid derivative	Fruits
Minerals	Potassium, calcium, magnesium ,sulfur, cadmium, phosphor, lead, titanium, vanadium, copper, silicon, barium, chromium, lithium, brome, aluminum, chloride, manganese, iron, sodium, zinc, strontium, and nitrogen	Fruits

Table 1.
General reported phyto-constituents of Rhus coriaria *and their parts of plant [12–22].*

7. Health promoting activities of *Rhus coriaria*

Rhus coriaria is an important flavoring spice with a wide range of health promoting activities (**Figure 3**). The plant exhibits antimicrobial, antioxidant, hypoglycemic, hypolipidimic, antimutagenic, antimigratory and anti-ischemic activities which are presented below.

7.1 Antimicrobial activities

Rhus coriaria poses antimicrobial activity against various bacterial and fungal species. Radmehr and Abdolrahimzade revealed the effectiveness of ethanol extract of sumac decreasing the minced meat total microbial count and salmonella, in which a potential antimicrobial significance was shown compared to controls [23]. Motaharinia et al. also examined the plant extract's antibacterial activity against *Brucella*, in which the MZG (mean zone of growth) inhibition for *Rhus coriaria* containing disks of 40 mg/ml was 22.55 mm, and MIC (minimum inhibitory concentration) of 3.26 mg/ml, while the MBC (minimum bactericidal concentration) was 9.03 mg/ml [24]. Furthermore, Shabir demonstrated an important *Rhus coriaria* fruit methanolic extract antibacterial activity against four different bacteria *Bordetella bronchiseptica*, *Bacillus pumilus*, *Staphylococcus epidermidis*, and *Klebsiella pneumonia*, utilizing agar well-diffusion method [10]. Kırmusaoğlu et al. evaluated in their study the *Rhus coriaria* antibacterial effect on the *Staphylococcus aureus* biofilm formation where significant differences between varying concentrations of extracts on several strains of methicillin resistant/sensitive *Staphylococcus aureus* were observed leading to the dose-related plant extracts diminishes the slime formation noted in bacteria with a clue that reduction of the biofilm formation which is a cornerstone playing factor in staphylococcal infections can be done with them [25]. Ali-Shtayeh et al. compared in their study the antimicrobial activity of *Rhus coriaria* among the 50 Palestinian medicinal plants against acne vulgaris, It was revealed from their result that the ethanolic extract of *Rhus coriaria* show a hard evidence inhibitory effect and found to be between the main active plant

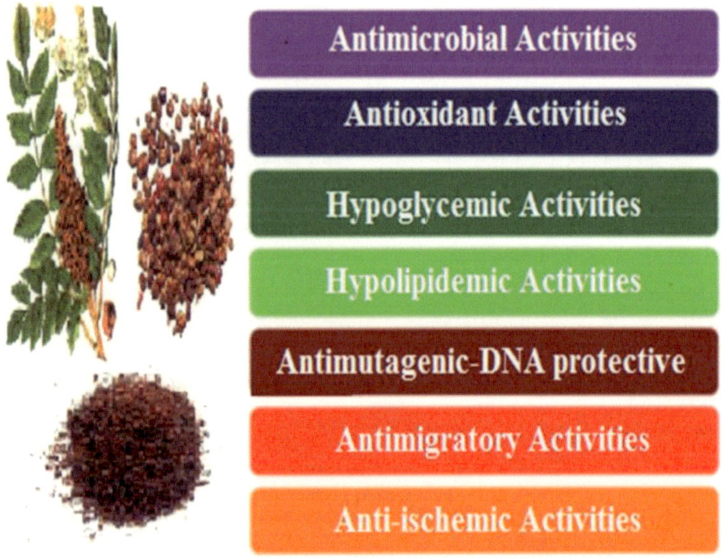

Figure 3.
Different health promoting activities of Rhus coriaria.

extracts against most bacterial strains tested including, *P. acnes*, and Gram-negative strains of aerobic bacteria [26]. Raodah et al. studied the *Rhus coriaria* extracts antimicrobial activity against three Gram-negative and three Gram-positive strains. The *Bacillus subtilis* was the most sensitive Gram-positive with MIC of 0.5 mg/ml, while higher concentrations of sumac were needed against Gram-negative bacteria with extracts concentrations ranging 10–20 mg/ml. Among bacteria, the inhibitory effects were shown to have positive relationship as an increased of *Rhus coriaria* fruit extracts concentration from 0.1 to 20 mg/ml lead to increasing the inhibitory effect [27]. It is valuable to mentioning that in vitro antimicrobial activity of *Rhus coriaria* extracts has been strongly suggested to the presence of tannins [28].

From another point of view, studies achieved on antifungal activity revealed that the alcohol extract of *Rhus coriaria* own a high antifungal activity to *Candida albicans* which is contributed to presence of coriariaoic acid, coriorianaphthyl ether and coriarianthracenyl ester in plant seeds [18, 29].

7.2 Antiviral activity

Monavari et al. manifested in their study that the *Rhus coriaria* aqueous extract show a potentially activity against viruses like adenovirus type 5 and HSV-1 at non-toxic concentration [30]. This activity related to presence of biflavones in *Rhus coriaria* leaves and fruits [5].

7.3 Antioxidant activity

Several studies have proven antioxidant activity of *Rhus coriaria*. Shafiei et al. studied the antioxidants and free radical scavengers as well as lipid peroxidation inhibition effects of methanol *Rhus coriaria* fruits and also indicated chronic diseases prevention such as atherosclerosis by the plant extract [31]. Aliakbarlu et al. demonstrated in their study the antioxidant potential ability of *Rhus coriaria* aqueous extract among other spices. Their study outcomes revealed that the aqueous extracts of the plant exhibit one of the highest antioxidant potential among the extracts studied [32]. *Rhus coriaria* is proved to have a significant antioxidative property due to its richness in phenolic compounds, especially, gallic acid and its derivatives [33]. Gabr et al. demonstrated that phenols derived from *Rhus coriaria* fruits had strong scavenging activities in vitro on β-carotene-linoleic acid and 2,2-diphenyl-1-picryl-hydrazyl-hydrate (DPPH) scavenging power assessment when compared to glycosides, alkaloids and terpenoids respectively [34].

The antioxidant capacities of ripened fruits of *Rhus coriaria* were estimated using DPPH and vanishment of dark violet color assays by Mahdavi et al. Their study revealed that *Rhus coriaria* had relatively high antioxidant capacity [8].

7.4 Hypoglycemic activity

The hypoglycemic activity of *Rhus coriaria* has been studied by numerous research groups. Mohammadi et al. studied the role of the ethanol extract of *Rhus coriaria* fruits upon glycaemia homeostasis and insulin resistance using alloxan induced diabetic rats as a model and significant hypoglycemic activity was observed [35]. Anwer et al. evaluated the effect of *Rhus coriaria* methanol extract on rats with diabetes mellitus non-insulin-dependent type. According to them, methanol extract of *Rhus coriaria* plant is able to improve insulin sensitivity, delaying the hyperinsulinemia onset and glucose intolerance [36]. In the first clinical trial, the effects of *Rhus coriaria* fruits in type 2 diabetic patients on the resistance of insulin, high sensitive CRP, malondialdehyde, and paraoxonase 1 activity were evaluated by Rahideh et al., presuming that daily intake of 3 g *Rhus coriaria* for 3 months may has a beneficial outcome on patients with diabetes mellitus decreasing their susceptibility for cardiovascular disease [37]. From all of above, the penta-galloylglucose (gallotannins) which was frequently conveyed in *Rhus coriaria* plant announced to have an antidiabetic effect, manifesting their activity by inhibiting the PTP1B enzyme [38].

7.5 Hypolipidimic activity

Many researches in this field indicated the positive effects of *Rhus coriaria* consumption on blood cholesterol level in animals and human beings. Their results showed the significant reduction in the triglyceride, cholesterol and low density lipoprotein-cholesterol (LDL) levels with protective effect against some risk factors caused by tissues fat overflow stress such as atherosclerosis, oxidative stress and hepatic enzymes dysfunction [31, 39–41].

7.6 Anti-mutagenic and DNA protective activity

Chakraborty et al. suggested the strong *Rhus coriaria* DNA migration reduction after 30% H_2O_2 treated cells. Endogenous production of oxidized pyrimidines and purines due to DNA-migration also decreased significantly by 36 and 52% respectively, especially in hepatic and lymphocyte damage which was the most significant decrease as the *Rhus coriaria* exhibit a protection capability against genotoxic carcinogens that are degraded by specific enzymes, specifically the GST (glutathione S-transferase), GST-α and GST-π which were enhanced by 40, 52 and 26% sequentially [33].

7.7 Anti-migratory activity

Zargham and Zargham demonstrated anti-migratory activity of *Rhus coriaria* fruits extract on rat carotid vascular smooth muscle cells using transmembrane migration assay. The biological assay showed that *Rhus coriaria* extracts considerable vascular smooth cell migration reduction by 62%, thus owning a strong anti-migratory potential, with a possible atheroprotective activity [42].

7.8 Anti-ischemic activities

The cardiovascular protective effect of *Rhus coriaria* leaves extracts was evaluated by measuring different factors such as RFS (free radical scavenging), TNF-α (tissue necrosis factor-α) inhibition, cyclooxygenase pathway activation and NO (nitric oxide) endothelial synthase activation in isolated rabbit heart and thoracic aorta preparations by Baretta et al. Their results suggest that *Rhus coriaria* possesses interesting substances (hydrolysable gallotannins) which act as anti-ischemic agents [43].

The neuroprotective and anti-neuroinflammatory properties of *Rhus coriaria* ethanol fruits extract was assessed against ischemic optic neuropathy in mice by Khalilpour et al. with outcomes providing a hard evidence scientific cornerstone for the neuroprotective activity of the ethanol *Rhus coriaria*, identifying linoleic acid as one of the main constituents responsible for such effect and leading the way for new treatment windows for optic neuropathy [44].

8. Applications of *Rhus coriaria* in food industrial safety and technology

There is a rising care for plant extracts investment in lipid oxidation control by natural preservatives in food industry as till now collected data goes with the application of *Rhus coriaria* as an oily foods natural antioxidant [45]. The plant extract had been used to enhance sausage total quality by preventing lipid oxidation, as it is more effective when compared with BHT (butylated hydroxytoluene) that has a carcinogenic and toxic properties, plant extract enhances the parameters of the fermented sausage quality [46]. Aqueous extracts of *Rhus coriaria* exhibit a powerful antibacterial activity with antioxidant power against pathogenic food-borne bacteria assuming their use as effective and natural industrial food preservatives [32], and these are also very useful delaying the food taste and aspect deterioration by the oxidative process [46].

An Italian study, Perna et al. had cogitate the sumac leafs powder application as a fortifier in the yogurt milk of goat taking the advantage of its antioxidant property. The *Rhus coriaria* goat milk fortified yogurt revealed a considerable increase in total phenolic compounds as compared with non- fortified goat milk yogurt. This raise the potential capability of using goat milk for the commercial production of the fermented fortified products allowing the evolution of nutraceutical fortified foods [47].

The antimicrobial growth properties of extracts in food are similar to the synthetic ones commonly used in food industry for the prevention of food microbiological degradation with quality maintenance and shelf life for more time [48].

The food additives were banned in many countries manufacturing and trading legislations, thus making the *Rhus coriaria* extracts one of the good alternatives for food decontamination compensating for banned synthetic and chemical antimicrobials used due to its properties of low prices, natural and as a safer alternative product increasing the shelf life and maintaining its quality with a good color in the score of sensory evaluation in the poultry processing [49]. Also the pure extract powder of the *Rhus coriaria* added carrier (maltodextrin) had been developed for spray drying [50]. Sumac had been used in feed additive in laying and broiler chicken to improve their quality [51].

Rhus coriaria use as colorant, as the sumac anthocyanins (main phenolic compound) are considered one of the pigmenting compounds in it with stability, are increased by intermolecular pigmentation after other polyphenolic addition interacting without covalent bond formation with the molecules preventing the nucleophilic attack by water molecule, making a more stable water mixed colorant agent extract [52].

9. Applications of *Rhus coriaria* in dentistry

Rhus coriaria is documented by many researchers to be a very food industry versatile material that is used in many fields leading the way for its use in other industries because of its components in the powder, aqueous and methanolic extracts that can be integrated in a wide ranged industrial fields to treat steel greenish color inhibition in moist environment like that in the mouth. This phenomenon attributed to specific ingredients found in sumac, which have the capability to adsorb with the steel metal ions forming ferrous organic molecule complexes [53]. Furthermore, this property of *Rhus coriaria* has a role in the medicinal applications such as a natural anticariogenic in the dentistry, as the aqueous extract has the ability to reduce the orthodontic wire bacterial biofilm formed on by the pathogenic bacterial species like: *Streptococcus sanguinis, Streptococcus sobrinus, Streptococcus salivarius, Streptococcus mutans* and *Enterococcus faecalis* [54]. *Rhus coriaria* also has the ability to decrease dental biofilm formation by *Streptococcus mutans* through the three GTF genes down-regulation without the suppression of the buccal bacteria growth [55].

10. Conclusions

Rhus coriaria is an important resourceful plant (Magical spice) in modern era due to its promising functional ingredients for nutraceuticals potential sources with various desirable medicinal properties and bioactivities with a reliable application of *Rhus coriaria* pharmacology and functional food preservative industries. There is consensus about its broad spectrum of biological activities as evident from this chapter. It possesses a broad range of phytochemical constituents such as hydrolysable tannins, phenolic acids, conjugated phenolic acids, anthocyanins, flavonoids, organic acids, coumarins, xanthones, terpenoids, steroids and essential oils demonstrated that it possess antimicrobial, antioxidant, hypoglycemic, hypolipidimic, antimutagenic, antimigratory and anti-ischemic activities. Overall contradicting evidence exist on the role of *Rhus coriaria* as a magical spice in the food industry as do for pharmaceuticals, playing a role that needs further delineation with encouraging evidence for its modulation needing further elucidation in human studies getting use of its synergizing effects in multiple fields making usefulness of its properties.

Author details

Thukaa Zuhair Abdul-Jalil
Department of Pharmacognosy, College of Pharmacy, University of Baghdad, Baghdad, Iraq

*Address all correspondence to: aljas_dadid@yahoo.com

References

[1] El-Sohaimy SA. Functional foods and nutraceuticals-modern approach to food science. World Applied Sciences Journal. 2012;**20**(5):691-708

[2] Upadhyay E, Almass AA, Dasgupta N. Assessment of occupational health hazards due to particulate matter originated from spices. International Journal of Environmental Research and Public Health. 2019;**16**(1519):1-13

[3] Sachan AK, Kumar S, Kumari K, Singh D. Medicinal uses of spices used in our traditional culture: Worldwide. Journal of Medicinal Plants Studies. 2018;**6**(3):116-122

[4] AL-Maa'thidy AM. A systematic study of the genus *Rhus* L. (Anacardiaceae) in Iraq. Al-Rafidain Science Journal. 2006;**10**:100-114

[5] Abu-Reidah IM, Jamous RM, Ali-Shtayeh MS. Phytochemistry, pharmacological properties and industrial applications of *Rhus coriaria* L. (sumac). Jordan Journal of Biological Sciences. 2014;**7**(4):233-244

[6] Sakhr K, El Khatib S. Physiochemical properties and medicinal, nutritional and industrial applications of Lebanese sumac (Syrian sumac-*Rhus coriaria*): A review. Heliyon. 2020;**6**:1-9

[7] Ahmad H, Ahmad F, Hasan I, Ahmad SH. Unani description of Sumaq (*Rhus coriaria* Linn.) and its scientific report. Global Journal of Medical Research. 2013;**13**(7):75-78

[8] Mahdavi S, Hesami B, Sharafi Y. Antimicrobial and antioxidant activities of Iranian sumac (*Rhus coriaria* L.) fruit ethanolic extract. Journal of Applied Microbiology and Biochemistry. 2018;**2**(25):1-5

[9] Asgarpanah J, Saati S. An overview on phytochemical and pharmacological properties of *Rhus coriaria* L. Research Journal of Pharmacognosy. 2014;**1**(3):47-54

[10] Shabbir A. *Rhus coriaria* Linn, a plant of medicinal, nutritional and industrial importance: A review. The Journal of Animal and Plant Sciences. 2012;**2**(2):505-512

[11] Lev E, Amar Z. "Fossils" of practical medical knowledge from medieval Cairo. Journal of Ethnopharmacology. 2008;**119**:24-40

[12] Abu-Reidah IM, Ali-Shtayeh MS, Jamous RM, Roman DA, Carretero AS. HPLC-DAD-ESI-MS/MS screening of bioactive components from *Rhus coriaria* L. (sumac) fruits. Food Chemistry. 2015;**166**:179-191

[13] Regazzoni L, Arlandini E, Garzon D, Santagati NA, Beretta G, Maffei FR. A rapid profiling of gallotannins and flavonoids of the aqueous extract of *Rhus coriaria* L. by flow injection analysis with high-resolution mass spectrometry assisted with database searching. Journal of Pharmaceutical and Biomedical Analysis. 2013;**72**:202-207

[14] Kossah R, Nsabimana C, Zhang H, Chen W. Optimization of extraction of polyphenols from Syrian sumac (*Rhus coriaria* L.) and Chinese sumac (*Rhus typhina* L.) fruits. Research Journal of Phytochemistry. 2010;**4**:146-153

[15] Kirby CW, Wu T, Tsao R, McCallum JL. Isolation and structural characterization of unusual pyranoanthocyanins and related anthocyanins from Staghorn sumac (*Rhus typhina* L.) via UPLC-ESI-MS, 1H, 13C, and 2D NMR spectroscopy. Phytochemistry. 2013;**94**:284-293

[16] Gabr SA, Alghadir AH. Phytochemical analysis and in vitro

antifungal activities of bioactive fractions from leaves of *Rhus coriaria* (SUMAC). Journal of Pure and Applied Microbiology. 2015;**9**:559-565

[17] Ünver A, Özcan MM. Fatty acid composition of seed and pericarp of sumac (*Rhus coriaria* L.) grown wild in different regions of Turkey. Journal of Food, Agriculture and Environment. 2010;**8**:31-33

[18] Singh O, Ali M, Akhtar N. New antifungal aromatic compounds from the seeds of *Rhus coriaria* L. International Research Journal of Pharmacy. 2011;**2**(1):188-194

[19] Morshedlooa MR, Maggib F, Nekoc HT, Aghdamd MS. Sumac (*Rhus coriaria* L.) fruit: Essential oil variability in Iranian populations. Industrial Crops and Products. 2018;**111**:1-7

[20] Farag MA, Fayek NM, Abou Reidah I. Volatile profiling in *Rhus coriaria* fruit (sumac) from three different geographical origins and upon roasting as analyzed via solid-phase microextraction. Peer Journal. 2018;**5121**:1-16

[21] Shabana MM, El Sayed AM, Yousif MF, El Sayed AM, Sleem AA. Bioactive constituents from *Harpephyllum caffrum* Bernh and *Rhus coriaria* L. Pharmacognosy Magazine. 2011;**7**:298-306

[22] Kizil S, Turk M. Microelement contents and fatty acid compositions of *Rhus coriaria* L. and *Pistacia terebinthus* L. fruits spread commonly in the south eastern Anatolia region of Turkey. Natural Product Research. 2010;**24**:92-98

[23] Radmehr B, Abdolrahimzade M. Antimicrobial effects of sumac (*Rhus coriaria* L.) extract in minced meat. Planta Medica. 2009;**75**(1068):PJ152

[24] Motaharinia Y, Rezaee MA, Hazhir MS, Zandi F, Shapouri R, Hakhamaneshi MS, et al. Evaluation of the antibacterial activity of *Zataria multiflora* Boiss, *Rhus coriaria* L. (sumac), *Mentha piperita* L., and *Ocimum basilicum* L. extracts on *Brucella* strains isolated from brucellosis patients. Turkish Journal of Medical Sciences. 2012;**42**:816-822

[25] Kırmusaoğlu S, Yurdugul S, Kocoğlu E. Effects of fermented sumac on the formation of slime layer of *Staphylococcus aureus*. Balkan Medical Journal. 2012;**29**:84-87

[26] Ali-Shtayeh MS, Al-Assali AA, Jamous RM. Antimicrobial activity of Palestinian medicinal plants against acne-inducing bacteria. African Journal of Microbiology Research. 2013;**7**:2560-2573

[27] Raodah M, Al-Ali AZH, Faleeha HH. The antioxidant and antimicrobial of Syrian sumac (*Rhus coriaria*) fruit extracts. Journal of Natural Science Research. 2014;**4**(11):36-40

[28] Rashid TS, Sijam K, Kadir J, Saud HM, Awla HK, Zulperi D, et al. Screening for active compounds in *Rhus coriaria* L. crude extract that inhibit the growth of *Pseudomonas syringae* and *Ralstonia solanacearum*. Indian Journal of Agricultural Research. 2016;**50**(1):15-21

[29] Ertürk Ö. Antibacterial and antifungal effects of alcoholic extracts of 41 medicinal plants growing in Turkey. Czech Journal of Food Sciences. 2010;**28**:53-60

[30] Monavari HR, Hamkar R, Norooz-Babaei Z, Adibi L, Noroozi M, Ziaei A. Antiviral effect assay of twenty five species of various medicinal plants families in Iran. Indian Journal of Medical Microbiology. 2007;**1**(2):49-59

[31] Shafiei M, Nobakht M, Moazzam AA. Lipid-lowering effect of *Rhus coriaria* L. (sumac) fruit extract in hypercholesterolemic rats. Pharmazie. 2011;**66**:988-992

[32] Aliakbarlu J, Mohammadi S, Khalili S. A study on antioxidant potency and antibacterial activity of water extracts of some spices widely consumed in Iranian diet. Journal of Food Biochemistry. 2013;**38**:159-166

[33] Chakraborty A, Ferk F, Simić T, Brantner A, Dušinská M, Kundi M, et al. DNA-protective effects of sumac (*Rhus coriaria* L.), a common spice: Results of human and animal studies. Mutation Research, Fundamental and Molecular Mechanisms of Mutagenesis. 2009;**661**:10-17

[34] Gabr SA, El-Metwally MM, AL-Ghadir AH. Antioxidant and antibacterial active constituents of *Rhus coriaria*. Biotechnology. 2014;**13**:37-45

[35] Mohammadi S, Kouhsari Montasser S, Feshani Monavar A. Antidiabetic properties of the ethanolic extract of *Rhus coriaria* fruits in rats. DARU Journal of Pharmaceutical Sciences. 2010;**18**:270-275

[36] Anwer T, Sharma M, Khan G, Iqbal M, Ali MS, Alam MS, et al. *Rhus coriaria* ameliorates insulin resistance in non-insulin-dependent diabetes mellitus (NIDDM) rats. Acta Poloniae Pharmaceutica. Drug Research. 2013;**70**:861-867

[37] Rahideh ST, Shidfar F, Khandozi N, Rajab A, Hosseini SP, Mirtaher SM. The effect of sumac (*Rhus coriaria* L.) powder on insulin resistance, malondialdehyde, high sensitive C-reactive protein and paraoxonase 1 activity in type 2 diabetic patients. Journal of Research in Medical Sciences: The Official Journal of Isfahan University of Medical Sciences. 2014;**19**:933-938

[38] Baumgartner RR, Steinmann D, Heiss EH, Atanasov AG, Ganzera M, Stuppner H, et al. Bioactivity-guided isolation of 1,2,3,4,6-penta-O-galloyl-d-glucopyranose from *Paeonia lactiflora* roots as a PTP1B inhibitor. Journal of Natural Products. 2010;**73**:1578-1581

[39] Setorki M, Rafieian M, Heidarian E, Ghatreh K, Shahinfard N, Ansari R, et al. Effect of *Rhus coriaria* consumption with high cholesterol food on some atherosclerosis risk factors in rabbit. Journal of Babol University of Medical Sciences. 2012;**14**:38-45

[40] Rouhi-Boroujeni H, Mosharraf S, Gharipour M, Asadi-Samani M, Rouhi-Boroujeni H. Anti-hyperlipidemic effects of sumac (*Rhus coriaria* L.): Can sumac strengthen anti-hyperlipidemic effect of statins? Der Pharmacia Lettre. 2016;**8**(3):143-147

[41] Nagib RM. Hypolipidemic effect of sumac (*Rhus coriaria* L) fruit powder and extract on rats fed high cholesterol diet. Bulletin of the National Nutrition Institute of the Arab Republic of Egypt. 2017;**50**:75-98

[42] Zargham H, Zargham R. Tannin extracted from sumac inhibits vascular smooth muscle cell migration. The Medical Journal of Malaysia. 2012;**11**:119-123

[43] Baretta G, Rossoni G, Santagati NA, Facino RM. Anti-ischemic activity and endothelium dependent vasorelaxant effect of hydrolysable tannins from the leaves of *Rhus coriaria* (sumac) in isolated rabbit heart and thoracic aorta. Planta Medica. 2009;**75**:1482-1488

[44] Khalilpour S, Behnammanesh G, Suede F, Ezzat MO, Muniandy J, Tabana Y, et al. Neuroprotective and

anti-inflammatory effects of *Rhus coriaria* extract in a mouse model of ischemic optic neuropathy. Biomedicine. 2018;**6**(48):1-13

[45] Özcan M. Antioxidant activities of rosemary, sage, and sumac extracts and their combinations on stability of natural peanut oil. Journal of Medicinal Food. 2003;**6**:267-270

[46] Bursal E, Koksal E. Evaluation of reducing power and radical scavenging activities of water and ethanol extracts from sumac (*Rhus coriaria* L.). Food Research International. 2011;**44**:2217-2221

[47] Perna A, Simonetti A, Grassi G, Gambacorta E. Effect of αS1-casein genotype on phenolic compounds and antioxidant activity in goat milk yogurt fortified with *Rhus coriaria* leaf powder. Journal of Dairy Science. 2018;**101**:7691-7701

[48] Obais AO, Alshouk AM, Jaafar KA. The antibacterial effect of sumac and myrtle extracts on the bacteria causative of soft rot disease in potatoes. Journal of University of Babylon. 2013;**21**:1622-1632

[49] El Khatib S, Salame A. Sumac (*Rhus coriaria*) extracts to enhance the microbiological safety of the red meat. Food Science and Technology. 2019;7(4):41-52

[50] Caliskan G, Nur Dirim S. The effects of the different drying conditions and the amounts of maltodextrin addition during spray drying of sumac extract. Food and Bioproducts Processing. 2013;**91**:539-548

[51] Salih YG, Gurbuz Y. Sumac (*Rhus coriaria* L.) and ginger (*Zingiber officinale*) as feed additive in poultry nutrition. KSU Journal of Natural Sciences. 2015;**18**:44-46

[52] Dabas D. Polyphenols as colorants. Advances in Food Technology and Nutritional Sciences—Open Journal. 2016;**2**:S1-S6

[53] Anaee R, Abdullah H, Tareq M. Sumac extract as green inhibitor for steel in seawater. International Journal of Scientific Research in Science, Engineering and Technology. 2016;**2**:353-358

[54] Dastjerdi E, Sarmast Z, Abdolazimi Z, Mahboubi A, Amdjadi P, Kamalinejad M. Effect of *Rhus coriaria* L. water extract on five common oral bacteria and bacterial biofilm formation on orthodontic wire. Iranian Journal of Microbiology. 2014;**6**:269-275

[55] Dastjerdi E, Monadi E, Khalighi H, Torshabi M. Down-regulation of glycosyl transferase genes in *Streptococcus mutans* by *Punica granatum* L. flower and *Rhus coriaria* L. fruit water extracts. Iranian Journal of Pharmaceutical Research. 2015;**15**:513-519

Chapter 5

An Overview of Genus *Zanthoxylum* with Special Reference to Its Herbal Significance and Application

Gyanmani Ekka, Shailesh Kumar Jadhav and Afaque Quraishi

Abstract

The plants of genus *Zanthoxylum* are effectually utilized in conventional and present-day medicine system to fight many diseases and disorders like pain, seizures, inflammation, cancer, liver and heart malady. Many of its plants—trees and shrubs, are citrus in nature, with curative antimicrobial, antihelminthic, antipyretic, and antiviral activities. More than 100 of its plant species have been identified and recorded for their potential as an herb in modern pharmacopeia. The species of this genus also have potent ethno-pharmacological significance. Many medicinal secondary metabolites like terpenoids, flavonoids, and alkaloids have also been profiled in many *Zanthoxylum* species. Additionally, fruit of many of the species is also significantly utilized as a major spice under the name "Sichuan pepper" in many countries like China and India. Thus, this unique blend of herb and spice characteristic of the genus needs a detailed description. This chapter highlights the major significant discoveries in the recent decade in this genus, which can add a step in the way of development of herbal medicines. Documentation of such medicinal plants may aid in derivation of plant-based medicines, which is the demand of the hour.

Keywords: cancer, herb, herbal, Sichuan pepper, *Zanthoxylum*

1. Introduction

Herbal or phyto-based medicines are in the mainstream of present pharmacological world [1]. Nearly two-thirds of the medicines throughout the world is plant based, the rest being the conventional ones [2]. The main reasons behind the preference of herbal drugs over the synthetic ones are that they have negligible side effects, are cost-effective, and easily available [3]. Also, the knowledge of herbal sources has led to the formation of base for many modern medicines. Some examples mentioned by Vickers and Zellman [4] are aspirin taken from willow bark, digoxin from foxglove, and morphine from opium poppy. Many researchers have also stated the development of resistance to allopathic drugs after a long medicament leading to becoming ineffective [5]. Thus, a documentation of medicinal plants and its herbal aspect becomes the first step toward a "botanical healing."

IntechOpen

2. *Zanthoxylum* genus

Zanthoxylum genus, belonging to family Rutaceae, comprises of aromatic, therapeutic deciduous shrubs and tree species [6]. Most of the plants in this genus are characterized by the presence of a strong lemon like odor, and prickly spines in the world [7]. The plant is mostly found in the South and Southeast Asian regions at an altitude of 1300–2500 m [7–9]. It is a plant of the warm temperate climate [10]. The benefits of this genus vary from healing common problems like toothache, gum problems, stomach ache, cough, cold, fever, dyspepsia, expulsion of roundworms, and in the treatment of fatal disease like cancer [11–16]. It is an anti-inflammatory, antinociceptive, antifertility, adipogenic, hepatoprotective agent; it also has the special ability to improve speaking power, reducing rheumatism, arthritis, asthma, skin diseases, abdominal pain, anorexia, ataxia, and purifying the blood [12, 15, 17–24]. The plant has phytomolecules that display insecticidal, antiparasitic, nematicidal, larvicidal, and fungicidal activities [13, 15, 25–29].

3. *Zanthoxylum* as herbal medicine in ancient pharmacology

Several species under *Zanthoxylum* genus have been used by various regions of the world since ancient times for benefits of mankind and their live stocks [5, 30, 31]. *Z. liebmannianum* bark is used for removal of parasites in Mexico [32]. For malaria, *Z. rhoifolium,* [33, 34] and *Z. acutifolium* [5] have been preferred from this genus. Nyishi tribe of India utilizes *Z. armatum* fruit, seed and bark in a traditional "Honyur" mix to treat stomach disorder, fever, and cholera, respectively [10]. *Z. chiloperene* var. angustifolium Engl. is also known as an antiparasitic agent in Paraguay [35]. *Z. integrifolium* bark is utilized by YaMei and Lanyu indigenous tribes of Taiwan, to treat dyspepsia and fever [5]. Freitas et al. [36] has reported antitumor and colitis-relief in *Z. rhoifolium* Lam. *Z. monophyllum* has found a place in the Venezulan medicine for treating jaundice, and ophthalmia [5]. Roots of *Z. zanthoxyloides* have been used to treat sickle cell anemia [37]. *Z. alatum* has been used for treatment of diabetes, toothaches, and abnormal cell growth [38].

4. *Zanthoxylum* as herbal medicine in modern pharmacology

4.1 Anticancerous activity

Z. leprieurii and *Z. zanthoxyloides* inhibits cancerous activity of leukemia (HL60) and (MCF7) breast cancer cell line [39]. It also shows moderate anti-cancerous activity (MCF-7), liver (WRL-68), prostrate (PC-3) and colon ($CACO_2$) carcinoma cell lines [37]. In another study, methanolic extract (ME) of the pericarp of *Z. armatum* revealed the presence of compounds ZP-amide A, C, D, E, hydroxyl α and β sanshool, and Timuramide A, B, C and D [9]. All these compounds inhibited the growth of mouse glioma cells that were deficient of tumor suppressor genes NF1 homolog-Nf1, whereas only few compounds showed activity against cell lacking Trp 53—the genes responsible for encoding tumor suppressor gene p53, at a concentration that is nontoxic to the nontumor cells. *Z. alatum* Roxb. stem bark petroleum ether extract (PE) possesses various anticancerous lignans, namely sesamin, kobusin, and 4′0 demethyl magnolin [38]. Out of which 4′0 demethyl magnolin, which is a novel compound, gave the best anticancerous output against lungs (A549) and pancreatic (MIA-PaCa) cancer cell lines, in comparison to the standard docetaxel. *Z. armatum* dried root ethyl acetate extract (EAE) (a good antioxidant) and its two components flavonoids, apigenin and kaempferol-7-O-glucoside, also possess an anticancerous trait against A-549, MIA-PaCa, MCF-7, and $CACO_2$ cancer colon cell lines [40]. In an extensive study, the ME of leaf of *Z. armatum* induced apoptosis in cervical cancer cell lines (HeLA) at IC_{50} (60 μg/mL) through Caspase 3-independent and extracellular signal-regulated kinases (ERK)-dependent mitogen-activated protein kinases (MAPK) apoptosis pathways [41]. Karmakar et al. [42] demonstrated that at an IC_{50} value of 102.30 μg/mL, the ME of the leaves of *Z. armatum* exhibited toxicity against Ehrlich Ascites cancer cells. The toxic effect was attributed to the presence of phenol and flavonoid compounds in the plant extract. Karmakar et al. [43] stated that the ME of leaves of this plant are capable of apoptosis by regulation of bcl-2/bax protein expressions and DNA damage in cancer cells and determined the presence of flavonoids, rutin, myricetin, and quercetin in the methanolic extract as potent anticancerous phytochemicals. Zanthonitrile [{4-[(3-Methyl-2-buten-1-yl) oxy] phenyl}acetonitrile] isolated from the leaves of the plant eluted by hexane: ethyl acetate solvent has a cytotoxic effect on Ehrlich Ascites Cancer cells with an IC_{50} value of 57.28 μg/mL [44]. Aqueous extract (AE) of *Z. piperitum* De Candolle fruit induces c-Jun N-terminal kinase autophagic cell death in colorectal (DLD-1), hepatocarcinoma (HepG2), and $CACO_2$ cancer cell lines but not in A549, MCF7, and colon (WiDr) cells [45]. Alam et al. [46] demonstrated that ME and crude saponins from leaves, fruit, and bark of *Z. armatum* have a potential of exerting a cytotoxic effect on breast (MDA-MB-468, MCF-71) and colorectal cancer (Caco-21) cell lines using the mechanism of apoptosis. Another compound Tambulin, a flavonoid isolated from the fruit exhibited antiproliferative action on certain cancer cell lines like MCF-7, WRL-68, COLO-205, MDAMB-231, with an IC_{50} ranging from 37.96 to 48.7 μg/mL [45]. Three compounds isolated from *Z. zanthoxyloides* fruits ME, hesperidin, skimmianine, and sesamine, possess anticancerous activity up to some level against A549, MCF7, and PC3 cell lines [47]. Pang et al. [48] confirms the anti-proliferative activity of seed oil of *Z. bungeanum* Maxim. on melanoma (A375) cells by arresting G1 phase and inducing apoptosis. Component analysis revealed the presence of unsaturated fatty acid in the seed oil. The EAE fraction of the fruit of *Z. acanthopodium* has been found effective for breast cancer cell line (T47D) toxicity [49]. Another isolated compound scoparone, a coumarin from the fruit of *Z. leprieurii*, at an IC_{50} of 44.93 μg/mL can be used to design anticancerous agents against human HepG2, with the least amount of toxicity to normal Chang liver cell lines [49]. Fruit of *Z. acanthopodium* in n-hexane fraction is also, effectively anticancerous toward T47D cell line [50]. The possible mechanism for this is cell cycle inhibition, apoptosis induction, and downregulation of cyclin D1 activity. Geranyl acetate is present in the highest percentage in the effective fruit n-fraction.

4.2 Neuroprotectant activity

Nakamura et al. [51] has reported that *Z. bungeanum* could reduce scopolamine-induced dementia. Gx-50, an isolate of *Z. bungeanum* could also aid in Alzheimer's disease, PE of the same plant can act as an antidepressant [52]. This compound gx-50 has the ability to cross blood–brain barrier and stop the degradation of nerve cells. Qinbunamide isolated from pericarp of *Z. bungeanum* can activate the nerve growth factor to further activate neurite outgrowth at 20 μM concentration [53]. Three alkaloids berberine, chelerythrine, and columbamine isolated from chloroform extract of *Z. schreberi* inhibit cholinesterase and butyrylcholinesterase [51]. As these enzymes are responsible for breakdown of acetyl choline, their inhibition leads to increase in number of nerve messengers, especially helpful in case of Alzheimer's and myasthenia gravis.

4.3 Antiparasitic activity

Z. chiloperone leaves EO and one of its major component canthin-6-one, showed an inhibition of parasitic activity of *Trypanosoma cruzi* at 10 mg/kg of oral and subcutaneous dose in comparison to standard benznidazole (dose 50 mg/kg) [35]. ME of *Z. armatum* seeds, at a concentration of 50 mg/mL induced paralysis in *Pheretima posthuma* (test model) in lesser time than the reference drug piperazine citrate (10 mg/mL) [54]. *Z. armatum* methanolic leaves extract at the concentrations of 250–1000 μg/mL showed a moderate trypanocidal activity on blood parasite found both in humans and animals—*Trypanosoma evansi* in an *in vitro* condition utilizing mice cells as a model [28]. Hexane bark extract of *Z. heitzii* acts as an inhibitor of *P. falciparum* at an IC_{50} 0.050 μg/mL [55]. Dihydronitidine one of the major components of the extract also acts as an antimalarial compound at an IC_{50} value of 0.0089 μg/mL [55]. In another investigation, anti-leishmanial activity was seen in crude extract and its hexane fraction of *Z. armatum* fruit against *Leishmania major* [46]. The essential oil (EO) of *Z. monophyllum* leaves also possess acute toxicity against larvae of *Anopheles subpictus* (LC_{50} 41.50 μg/mL), *Aedes albopictus* (LC_{50} 45.35 μg/mL), and *Culex tritaeniorhynchus* (LC_{50} 49.01 μg/mL). Among its two major compounds Germacrene D-4-ol has better efficiency than α-Cadinol [56]. Also, The EO, along with Germacrene D-4-ol, and α-Cadinol, EO has very low toxicity against *Gambusia affinis,* an eradicator of malarial larvae. Costa et al. [57], has reported antiparasitic activity of three noval compounds (5,7,8-trimethoxy coumarin, syringaresinol, and dictamine, isolated from the ethanol extract (EE) of roots of *Z. tingoassuiba* against *Leishmania amazonensis* and *Trypanosoma cruzi*, similar to positive control benznidazole and amphotericin. The larval stage of *Schistosoma haematobium*, a bladder cancer causing parasite can be successfully eliminated by acridone compound arborinine, isolated from fruit of *Z. leprieurii* at an IC_{50} value of 6.98 μg/mL [57].

4.4 Antimicrobial activity

Bark EE of *Z. fagara*, *Z. elephantiasis,* and *Z. martinicense* presented antifungal activity against fungi prevalent in domestic animals—*Aspergillus flavus*, *A. niger*, *Candida albicans*, *Saccharomyces cerevisiae*, *Microsporum canis*, *Trichophyton mentagrophytes* [31]. Though, it was unable to inhibit bacteria like *Staphylococcus aureus*, *Escherichia coli*, *Klebsiella pneumonia*, and *Psuedomonas aeruginosa* [31]. Lipophilic leaf of *Z. armatum* extract was found effective against *Alternaria alternata* and *Curvularia lunata* [58]. The EE of the whole *Z. armatum* plant proved to be effective against *S. aureus* (7 mm zone of inhibition), *Bacillus subtilis* (23 mm the biggest zone of inhibition), *B. cereus* (6 mm zone of inhibition), and *B. thuringiensis* (1 mm zone of inhibition) [25]. Barkatullah et al. [18] reported a maximum inhibition of *Micrococcus luteus*, *Pasteurella multocida*, *E. coli,* and *B. subtilis* by the application of *Z. armatum* leaf EE. *Z. leprieurii* and *Z. xanthoxyloides* EO decreased the effective time required to deactivate 7log cfu/mL of *Salmonella enteritidis* [59]. Oxychelerythrine, a benzophenanthridine alkaloid extracted from the ME of roots of *Z. capense* Thunb. altered the sensitivity of *S. aureus* ATCC 6538 to tested antibiotics (erythromycin, oxacillin, and tetracycline) in a positive way by twofold [60]. According to Alam and Saqib [46], n-hexane, chloroform, and aqueous-methanol fraction of *Z. armatum* fruits are a potent antifungal source, especially against *Trichophyton longifusus*, *Microsporum canis*,

A. flavus, *Fusarium solani*. The presence of alkaloids may be the reason behind such activity. Chen et al. [61] has found antimicrobial activity in the leaves extract of *Z. bungeanum* Maxim. against *E. coli. K. pneumonia, P. aeruginosa, S. enteritidis, Listeria monocytogenes, C. albicans*. Mirza et al. [62] observed that *Z. armatum* aqueous leaves extract-derived copper oxide nanomaterials (100 μl) was more sensitive in all bacterial strains tested (*S. aureus, Streptococcus mutans, Streptococcus pyrogenes, Staphylococcus epidermidis, B. cereus, Corynebacterium xerosis, E. coli, K. pneumonia, P. aeruginosa,* and *Proteus vulgaris*) in comparison to its source plant extract (100 μl).

Potent tuberculosis plant: ME of *Z. leprieurii* at minimum inhibitory concentrations (MIC) of 47.5, 75.3 and 125.0 μg/mL inhibited rifampicin-resistant and isoniazid-resistant strains of *Mycobacterium tuberculosis,* respectively [63]. Hydroxy-1,3-dimethoxy-10-methyl-9-acridone, 1-hydroxy-3-methoxy-10-methyl-9-acridone, and 3-hydroxy-1, 5,6-trimethoxy-9-acridone isolated from the plant also exhibited potent inhibition of resistant strains [63].

4.5 Antiviral activity

Z. coreanum root extract at an IC_{50} of 1.0 μg/mL inhibited porcine epidemic diarrhea virus growth [5]. Moreover *Z. planispinum* also exhibited the similar activity at an IC_{50} of 6.4 and 7.5 μg/mL respectively. Patino et al. [5] also reported the anti-HIV activity of *Z. ailanthoides*, *Z. integrifoliolum,* and *Z. scandens*.

4.6 Antioxidant activity

Oxypeucedanin, a coumarin compound present in ME of roots of *Z. flavum* Vahi., possesses significant antioxidant activity with an IC_{50} value of 8.3 μg/mL in a dichloro-dihydro-fluorescein diacetate (DCFH-DA) assay [32]. Z. *armatum* fruit EE showed promising activity as a natural source of antioxidants [64]. According to their study, the bioactive compound responsible for such quenching action is flavonoids, especially quercetin. Moreover, the EE of its stem bark tested via 2,2′-diphenyl picrylhydrazyl (DPPH) free radical scavenging activity exhibited significant antioxidant activities [23]. DPPH radical scavenging activity was obtained in the sequence of ME of stems (IC_{50} 54.6 ± 2.9 μg/mL) > dichloromethane extract of stems (IC_{50} 4.7 ± 117.5 μg/mL) > EO of fruits (IC_{50} 5764.7 ± 6.5 μg/mL) of plant *Z. limonella* Alston [65]. Singh et al. [65] reported that the EO from the seeds of *Z. armatum* was a potent antioxidant. Ethyl acetate fraction and aqueous fraction of *Z. bungeanum* showed potent DPPH, 2,2′-azino-bis(3-ethylbenzothiazoline-6-sulfonic acid (ABTS) radical scavenging abilities and ferric-reducing antioxidant power (FRAP) [66]. The EO and its constituent oleoresins showed moderate antioxidant activity when evaluated by DPPH radical scavenging, Fe^{2+} chelating, ferric thiocyanate method, and different lipid peroxidation assays. Leaves extract of *Z. bungeanum* maxim "You Huajiao" variety from China possess DPPH and ABTS radical scavenging activity. It also possesses the reducing potent power (FRAP) [61]. A compound Ombuin isolated from the fruit of *Z. armatum* possessed antioxidant capacity [67]. Two new sesquiterpenoid glycosides, dihydrophaseic acid 4′-O-[6″-O-(4‴-hydroxy-3‴, 5‴-dimethoxy) benzoyl)]-b-D-glucopyranoside and dihydrophaseic acid 4′-O-[6″-O-(3‴-methoxy4‴-hydroxy) benzoyl)]-b-D-glucopyranoside, isolated from the ethanolic extract of stems of *Z. armatum* showed moderate scavenging activity in DPPH free radical assay with IC_{50} values of 241 and 264 μM, respectively [68]. Aqueous extract of leaves of *Z. armatum* and copper oxide nanoparticles derived from it were less effective in DPPH radical scavenging activity in comparison to L-ascorbic [40].

4.7 Anti-inflammatory activity

The crude extract of *Z. armatum* reduced thermal pain significantly at the concentrations of 100 and 400 mg/kg body weight in case of intraperitoneal (i.p.), in comparison to 30 mg/kg body weight i.p. of standard anti-inflammatory drug phenacetin [69]. Also, its root extract exhibited analgesic activity when compared to standard drug indomethacin (40 mg/kg body weight i.p.) [69]. The anti-inflammatory activity of EE of the stem bark of *Z. armatum* against paw edema in Wistar rats has also been observed by Sati et al. [23]. Thus, *Z. armatum* may be helpful in the treatment of pain and inflammation symptoms. Eight lignans that may be responsible for this curative quality, namely eudesmin, horsfieldin, fargesin, kobusin, sesamin, asarinin, planispine A, and pinoresinol-di-3,3-dimethylallyl, were recognized by HPLC analysis in its EE of stem and root [70]. Nine terpenylated coumarins, namely 7-[(E)30,70-dimethyl-60-oxo-20,70-octadienyl]oxy-coumarin, schinilenol, schinindiol, collinin, 7-[(E)-70-hydroxy-30,70-dimethy-locta-20,50-dienyloxy]-coumarin, 8-methoxyanisocoumarin, 7-(60R-hydroxy-30,70-dimethyl-20E,70-octadienyloxy)coumarin, (E)-4-methyl-6-(coumarin-70-yloxy)hex-4-enal, and aurapten, along with a 4-quinolone alkaloid and integrifoliodiol, isolated from the leaves of *Z. schinifolium* by α-glucosidase inhibitory effect showed anti-inflammatory activity [71]. EO from fruits of *Z. coreanum* Nakai inhibited both the IgE-antigen complex and IL4 production in RBL-2H3 mast cells showing anti-inflammatory activity [60]. 2α-methyl-2β-ethylene-3β-isopropyl-cyclohexan-1β, 3α-diol and phenol-O-β-D-arabinopyranosyl-4′-(3″,7″,11″,15″-tetramethyl) hexadecan-1″-oate noval compound isolated from the methanolic extract of *Z. armatum* fruit exhibited anti-inflammatory activity by inhibiting pro-inflammatory cytokines like TNF-α and IL-6 in peritoneal macrophages at the concentration of 5 and 10 μg/mL [72].

4.8 Antihyperglycemic activity

Z. armatum bark ME exhibits anti-hyperglycemic activity against streptozotocin-induced diabetic rats at 200 and 400 mg/kg concentration [73]. Stem bark AE of *Z. chalybeum* Engl. displayed anti-hyperglycemic activity at 10, 100, and 1000 mg/kg body weight concentration against streptozotocin-induced diabetic rats [74]. n-Butanol fraction of *Z. alatum* EE inhibits can inhibit protein tyrosine phosphatase-1B and stimulates glucose uptake in C2CL2 myotubes in streptozotocin-induced diabetic rats [75]. *Z. armatum* aqueous leaves extract the activity α amylase, and α and β glucosidase, thus, can act as an antidiabetic agent [75].

4.9 Insecticidal activity

Di-chloromethane extract of *Z. usambarense* bark displayed insecticidal activity against *Masca domestica* at 5000 g/ha, but its individual component could not produce any insecticidal results [70]. The EO contained sabinene, D-germacrene, β-mycrene, β-elemene and γ-elemene. The larvicidal potential of EO and its constituent from the seeds of *Z. armatum* were screened against three mosquito species, *Aedes aegypti*, *Anopheles stephensi*, and *Culex quinquefasciatus* [15]. Among these three species, *C. quinquefasciatus* showed the highest sensitivity at lowest concentration LC_{50} and LC_{95} at 49 and 146 ppm, respectively. However, linalool the most important constituent present at the maximum concentration (57%) in the EO failed to establish any significant larvicidal effect individually [15]. Hieu et al. [76] revealed that mixtures of *Z. armatum* seed oil (ZA-SO) and its constituents either alone (0.2 mg/cm^2) or as a binary mixture (0.01 + 0.99 mg/cm^2) with

Calophyllum inophyllum nut oil (CI-NO) can be potential repellents against stable fly, *Stomoxys calcitrans*. An aerosol of the mixture (ZA-SO-2.5% + CI-NO-2.5%) was also found effective as a repellent of stable fly. Among all its constituents tested, only methyl cinnamate exhibited a significant effect [77]. In a different study, three bioactive compounds—piperitone, myrtanol, and citronellal from *Z. armatum* seed oil were assessed for fumigant toxicity potency against stable fly with a simultaneous comparison of chlorpyrifos and dichlorvos, which are the organophosphorus insecticides [78]. The fumigant toxicity potential of seed oil and all three compounds according to the vapor phase assay was high with LC_{50} value 0.242–0.456 μg/cm^3, but their toxic level was five magnitudes below the organophosphorus insecticides, which reflects that *Z. armatum* may be further used as a bio-insecticide [78]. Additionally, constituents of EO-cuminaldehyde citronellal, neral, linalool, linalool oxide, terpinen-4-ol, 1,8-cineole, and piperitone induced a significant repellent behavior in the stable fly [76]. The *in vitro* insecticidal efficacy of the EE of the bark of the plant has been observed against mustard aphid *Lipaphis erysimi* at the concentrations of 0.5, 1.0, 1.5, and 2.0 mg/L [79]. After 24 h of spray at a concentration of 2.0 mg/L, 100% mortality of the aphid was there, proving that *Z. armatum* may be a good insecticide [79]. Nanoencapsulated EO of *Z. rhoifolium* leaves efficiently reduced the number of eggs and nymphs of *Bemisia tabaci* at 1–5% concentration [80]. Out of 32 constituents identified from the EE of *Z. armatum* twigs, 1,8-cineole piperitone, and limonene in particular were efficient as an insecticide against *Lasioderma serricorne* and *T. castaneum* [81]. While, in another study, the effect of *Z. armatum* leaves methanolic extract has been checked for antifeedant activity on the adults of "Red flour beetle"–*T. castaneum* [82]. Another study stated the effects of n-hexane, EE, and ME of leaves of *Z. armatum* on *Plutella xylostella*, diamondback moth [83]. In this investigation, the n-hexane fraction exhibited the best larvicidal activity at an LC_{50} value of 2988.6 ppm. Moreover, two compounds, particularly 2-undecanone and 2-tridecanone identified from the n-hexane fraction of leaf extract of *Z. armatum* through GC–MS analysis, which may be responsible for the larvicidal activity [83]. Egg laying capacity of *Bemisia tabaci*, a major tomato pest, can be reduced (85–98%) by using EO of *Z. rhoifolium* and *Z. riedelianum* at 1.0–2.0% concentration [84].

4.10 Nematicidal activity

EO of *Z. armatum* fruit showed more than 90% nematicidal activity 5 mg/mL concentration against *Bursaphelenchus xylophilus*, whereas its components methyl trans cinnamate and ethyl trans cinnamate also exhibited 100% activity at 0.0625–2.0 and 0.25–2.0 mg/mL, respectively [85]. *Z. armatum* leaves AE (100–400 mg/kg body weight concentration) decreased the hatching ability of *Meloidogyne incognita* [13]. The leaves of *Z. armatum* also work as a nematicide on *M. incognita* if added directly in the soil at the concentrations of 8, 10, and 20 g/kg of soil [86].

4.11 Hepatoprotective activity

Glycoprotein isolates of *Z. piperitum* DC fruit inhibited hypoxanthine/xanthine oxidase [87]. It also decreased the level of lactate dehydroenase, thio barbituric acid, while increasing the level of antioxidant enzymes in carbon tetrachloride acute liver damage. The leaf EE of *Z. armatum* significantly decreased all the symptoms of hepatotoxicity in Wistar albino rats by normalizing the elevated levels of hepatic enzymes, which was induced by carbon tetrachloride [24]. It induced hepatoprotective activity at a concentration of 500 mg/kg of body weight in comparison to standard drug silymarin at a dose of 100 mg/kg body weight. This effect was there due to the radical scavenging activity of the phytochemicals, especially flavonoids present in the plant [24]. In a different study, the EE of bark of *Z. armatum* significantly expressed hepatoprotective activity at concentrations of 100, 200, and 400 mg/kg when administered orally in Wistar albino rats (where liver damage was instigated by paracetamol) by decreasing the levels of hepatic enzymes, bilirubin and at the same time increasing catalase, superoxide dismutase, and glutathione in comparison to silymarin [88]. In a recent study the ME at a dose of 500 mg/kg exhibited successful hepatoprotective activity with 66.87, 64.84, 67.95, 60.76, and 65.85% protection on aspartate aminotransferase, alanine aminotransferase, alkaline phosphatase, total bilirubin, and total protein enzyme levels of the liver, respectively in Wistar rats [89].

4.12 Gastroprotective activity

Z. rhoifolium Lam. stem bark EE prevents the formation of gastric lesions at 125–500 mg/kg dose by increasing enzymes like catalase (reduces oxidative stress) and also mucous secretion, nitric oxide (repair of gastrointestinal tract injury) [36]. It also helps in opening K_{ATP} channel to control H^+ pump and acid secretion. *Z. bungeanum* pericarp extract reduces the level of TNF-α, IL-1β, and IL-12 to reduce the inflammation in J774.1 colon cells [90]. Thus it can be utilized to treat ulcerative colitis.

4.13 Cardiovascular activity

Z. bungeanum EO at the concentration of 5, 10, and 20 mL/kg had a significant effect on deduction of cholesterol, hyperlipidemia, triglyceride, and low-density lipoprotein; it also aided in the induction of high-density lipoprotein [91]. The EO of *Z. bungeanum* also helped in relaxation of contracted aortic muscles by reducing calcium influx via calcium channels [90]. *Z. armatum* fruits hydroethanolic extract (dose administered—200 and 400 mg/kg body weight) succeeded in decreasing the elevated levels of cardiac diagnostic marker enzymes (aspartate aminotransferase, alanine aminotransferase, lactate dehydrogenase, creatine kinase-MB, troponin-T), lipid profile and antioxidants (enzymatic and nonenzymatic), to normal conditions. The results were comparable to a positive control verapamil, expected phytochemicals are yet to be identified [92].

4.14 Antiobesity activity

In a study, methyl cinnamate, an important bioactive compound of the *Z. armatum* suppressed the intracellular lipid accumulation [20]. It was possible at a concentration of 25 μM through Ca^{2+}/calmodulin-dependent protein kinase kinase 2 (CaMKK2)-phospho AMP-activated protein kinase (AMPK) signaling pathway, by downregulating the adipogenic transcription factors, sterol regulatory element binding protein-1 (SREBP-1), peroxisome proliferator-activated receptor γ (PPARγ), and CCAAT/enhancer-binding protein α (C/EBPα), as well as inhibiting the activity of PPARγ and glycerol-3-phosphate dehydrogenase (GPDH) in 3 T3-L1 preadipocyte cells [20].

5. *Zanthoxylum* as spice

"Sichuan pepper" with its pungent odor and numbing taste belongs to the genus *Zanthoxylum* [93]. According to Ji et al. [94] five species of Zanthoxylum—*Z. armatum*, *Z. bungeanum*, *Z. shinifolim*, *Z. simulans*, *Z. piperitum,* are commonly considered as "spice" species of the family. Not only seeds, fruit, leaves, bark, and even root of this genus is used as spice in China, Japan, and Korea [95]. This pepper is used by the people of China to create a special "Mala" flavor, which literally refers to numbness and spiciness. More than hundred volatile compounds have been isolated, which are responsible for the unique spicy note and fragrance of this genus [96]. Some nonvolatile compounds have also been identified like alkylamides (sanshools, capsaicin) and polyphenolic compounds [97]. The genus has found a place in culinary as "five spice powder," in cosmetics, as well as in pharmaceutical too [98]. In cosmetics, the variable fragrance provided by the genus—sweet, spearmint, herbal, floral, fruity, rose, citrus—is of great significance [99]. This diversity is due to the presence of more than hundred volatile compounds like 1,8-cineole, 1-terpineol, 2,-nonenal, 2-tridecanone, α-elemol, α-pinene, β-pinene, geraniol, myrcene, neryl acetate, piperitone, rosefuran etc. [100]. The pungent property of the spice of this genus has been attributed to the presence of α-, β-, γ-δ-sanshool and hydroxyl α and β-sanshool [99]. In pharmacology the presence of polyphenolic compounds like flavonoids and glycosides make Sichuan pepper a good antioxidant and anti-inflammatory agent. Zhu et al. [98] has also reported the presence of antibacterial activity against both gram positive and negative bacteria in EO of *Z. bungeanum* fruit. EO of *Z. shinifolium* and *Z. piperitum* (broad spectrum) has been reported to have antiviral properties [94]. Most significantly, Sichuan pepper and its component sanshool amide have displayed inhibitory action on the formation of hetercyclic amines, which are carcinogenic to humans in beef grilling procedure [11, 101]. Utilization of analytical techniques to compare component analysis is lacking in the literature related to spice knowledge of the genus. Also according to Ji et al. [94] if the effect of heat (while cooking) is elaborated on the spice and its individual compound, it would be more beneficial to the herb and spice world.

6. Conclusion and future perspective

Zanthoxylum genus is a stockpile of medicinal plants brewing with therapeutic properties, as gathered from the above references of the recent decade. The readers can benefit with the traditional and current knowledge on the herbal aspect of several species *Z. acanthopodium, Z. acutifolium, Z. ailanthoides, Z. armatum, Z. bungeanum, Z. chalybeum, Z. chiloperone, Z. coreanum, Z. elephantiasis, Z. fagara, Z. flavum, Z. heitzii, Z. integrifoliolum, Z. leprieurii, Z. liebmannianum, Z. limonella, Z. martinicense, Z. monophyllum, Z. piperitum, Z. planispinum, Z. rhoifolium, Z. riedelianum, Z. scandens, Z. schinifolium, Z. schreberi, Z. tingoassuiba, Z. usambarense, Z. zanthoxyloides* to name a few, of this genus. The information can form the basis of research regarding drug formulations, conservation of medicinal plants, pharmacokinetics, and new drug discoveries, which are plant based in the future.

Author details

Gyanmani Ekka, Shailesh Kumar Jadhav and Afaque Quraishi*
School of Studies in Biotechnology, Pt. Ravishankar Shukla University, Raipur, India

*Address all correspondence to: drafaque13@gmail.com

References

[1] Kamboj VP. Herbal medicine. Current Science. 2000;**78**:35-39

[2] Newman DJ, Cragg GM. Natural products as sources of new drugs over the last 25 years. Journal of Natural Products. 2007;**70**:461-477

[3] Pal S, Shukla Y. Herbal medicine: Current status and the future. Asian Pacific Journal of Cancer Prevention. 2002;**4**:281-288

[4] Vickers A, Zollman C. ABC of complementary medicine: Herbal medicine. British Medical Journal. 1999;**319**:1050-1053

[5] Patino OJ, Prieto JA, Cuca LE. *Zanthoxylum* genus as potential source of bioactive compounds. In: Rasooli I, editor. Bioactive Compounds in Phytomedicine. London, United Kingdom: IntechOpen; 2012. DOI: 10.5772/26037

[6] Ahmad A, Misra LN, Gupta MM. Hydroxalk-(4Z)-enoic acids and volatile components from the seeds of *Zanthoxylum armatum*. Journal of Natural Products. 1993;**56**:456-460

[7] Datt G, Chauhan JS, Ballabha R. Influence of pre-sowing treatments on seed germination of various accessions of Timroo (*Zanthoxylum armatum* DC.) in the Garhwal Himalaya. Journal of Applied Research on Medicinal and Aromatic Plants. 2017;**7**:89-94

[8] Alam F, Saqib QN. Pharmacognostic study and development of quality control parameters for fruit, bark and leaf of *Zanthoxylum armatum* (Rutaceae). Ancient Science of Life. 2015;**34**:147-155

[9] Devkota KP, Wilson J, Henrich CJ, McMahon JB, Reilly KM, Beutler JA. Isobutylhydroxyamides from the pericarp of Nepalese *Zanthoxylum armatum* inhibit *NF1*-defective tumor cell line growth. Journal of Natural Products. 2013;**76**:59-63

[10] Shankar R, Rawat MS. Conservation and cultivation of threatened and high valued medicinal plants in north East India. International Journal of. Biodiversity and Conservation. 2013;**5**:584-591

[11] Kalia NK, Singh B, Sood RP. A new amide from *Zanthoxylum armatum*. Journal of Natural Products. 1999;**62**:311-312

[12] Kumar V, Kumar S, Singh B, Kumar N. Quantitative and structural analysis of amides and lignans in *Zanthoxylum armatum* by UPLC-DAD-ESI-QTOF-MS/MS. Journal of Pharmaceutical and Biomedical Analysis. 2014;**94**:23-29

[13] Mukhtar T, Kayani MZ, Hussain MA. Nematicidal activities of *Cannabis sativa* L. and *Zanthoxylum alatum* Roxb. Against *Meloidogyn incognita*. Industrial Crops and Products. 2013;**42**:447-453

[14] Thakur T, Trak TH, Tripathi J. Ethnomedicinal use of some of the plants of Udhampur district of Jammu and Kashmir, India. Indian Journal of Applied and Pure Biology. 2017;**32**:293-300

[15] Tiwary M, Naik SN, Tewary DK, Mittal PK, Yadav S. Chemical composition and larvicidal activities of the essential oil of *Zanthoxylum armatum* DC. (Rutaceae) against three mosquito vectors. Journal of Vector Borne Diseases. 2007;**44**:198-204

[16] Waheed A, Mahmud S, Akhtar M, Nazir T. Studies on the components of essential oil of *Zanthoxylum armatum* by GC-MS. American Journal of Analytical Chemistry. 2011;**2**:258-261

[17] Barkatullah IM, Muhammad N. Evaluation of *Zanthoxylum armatum* DC for *in vitro* and *in vivo* pharmacological screening. African Journal of Pharmacy and Pharmacology. 2011;**5**:1718-1723

[18] Barkatullah IM, Muhammad N, Tahir L. Antimicrobial evaluation, determination of total phenolic and flavonoid contents in *Zanthoxylum armatum* DC. Journal of Medicinal Plant Research. 2012;**6**:2105-2110

[19] Bhatia H, Sharma YP, Manhas RK, Kumar K. Ethnomedicinal plants used by the villagers of district Udhampur, J & K. Journal of Ethnopharmacology. 2014;**151**:1005-1018

[20] Chen Y, Lee M, Hsu C, Wei C, Tsai Y. Methyl cinnamate inhibits adipocyte differentiation via activation of the caMKK2-AMPK pathway in 3T3 L1 preadipocytes. Journal of Agricultural and Food Chemistry. 2012;**60**:955-963

[21] Fatima A, Ahmad M, Zafar M, Yaseen G, Khan MPZ, Butt MA, et al. Ethnopharmacological relevance of medicinal plants used for treatment of oral diseases in Central Punjab-Pakistan. Journal of Herbal Medicine. 2017;**12**:88-110

[22] Guo T, Deng Y, Xie H, Yao C, Cai C, Pan S. Antinociceptive and anti-inflammatory activities of ethyl acetate fraction from *Z. armatum* in mice. Fitoterapia. 2011;**82**:347-351

[23] Sati SC, Sati MD, Raturi R, Badoni P, Singh H. Anti-inflammatory and antioxidant activities of *Zanthoxylum armatum* stem bark. Global Journal of Engineering Research. 2011;**11**:19-21

[24] Verma N, Khosa RL. Hepato-protective activity of leaves of *Z. armatum* DC. in CCL4 induced hepatotoxicity in rats. Indian Journal of Biochemistry and Biophysics. 2010;**47**:124-127

[25] Joshi B, Lekhak S, Sharma A. Antibacterial property of different medicinal plants: *Ocimum sanctum*, *Cinnamomum zeylanicum*, *Xanthoxylum armatum*, *Origanum majorana*. Kathmandu University Journal of Science, Engineering and Technology. 2009;**5**:143-150

[26] Ramanujam SN, Ratha BK. Effect of alcohol extract of a natural piscicide – Fruits of *Zanthoxylum armatum* DC. On Mg2+ - and Na+, K+ ATPase activity in various tissues of a freshwater air breathing fish, *Heteropneustes fossilis*. Aquaculture. 2008;**283**:77-82

[27] Raturi R, Badoni PP, Ballabha R. Insecticidal and fungicidal activities of stem bark of *Zanthoxylum armatum* (Rutaceae). World Journal of Pharmacy and Pharmaceutical Sciences. 2014;**3**:1838-1843

[28] Shaba P, Pandey NN, Sharma OP, Rao JR, Singh RK. Therapeutic effects of *Zanthoxylum alatum* leaves and *Eugenia caryophyllata* buds (fruits) against *Trypanosoma evansi*. Journal of Animal and Veterinary Advances. 2012;**2**:91-97

[29] Xu D, Zhuo Z, Wang R, Ye M, Pu B. Modeling the distribution of *Zanthoxylum armatum* in China with maxEnt modeling. Global Ecology and Conservation. 2019;**19**:e00691

[30] Adesina SK. The Nigerian *Zanthoxylum*: Chemical and biological values. African Journal of Traditional, Complementary, and Alternative Medicines. 2005;**2**:282-301

[31] Dieguez-Hurtado R, Garrido-Garrido G, Prieto-Gonzalez S, Iznaga Y, Gonzalez L, Molina-Torres J, et al. Antifungal activity of some Cuban *Zanthoxylum* species. Fitoterapia. 2003;**74**:384-386

[32] Ross SA, Sultana GNN, Burandt CL, ElSohly MA, Marais JPJ, Ferreira D. Syncaparmide, a new antiplasmodial

(+)-norepinephrine derivative from *Zanthoxylum syncarpum*. Journal of Natural Products. 2004;**67**:88-90

[33] Bertani S, Bourdy G, Landau I, Robinson JC, Esterre PH, Deharo E. Evaluation of French Guiana traditional antimalarial remedies. Journal of Ethnopharmacology. 2005;**98**:45-54

[34] Jullian V, Bourdy G, Georges S, Maurel S, Sauvain M. Validation of use of a traditional remedy from French Guiana, *Zanthoxylum rhoifolium* lam. Journal of Ethnopharmacology. 2006;**106**:348-352

[35] Ferreira ME, Cebrian-Torrejon G, Corrales AS, Vera De Bilbao N, Rolon M, Gomez CV, et al. *Zanthoxylum chiloperone* leaves extract: First sustainable Chagas disease treatment. Journal of Ethnopharmacology. 2011;**133**:986-993

[36] Freitas FFBP, Fernandes HB, Piauilino CA, Pereira SS, Carvalho KIM, Chaves MH, et al. Gastroprotective activity of *Zanthoxylum rhoifolium* lam in animal models. Journal of Ethnopharmacology. 2011;**137**:700-708

[37] Misra LN, Wouatsa NAV, Kumar S, Kumar V, Tchoumbougnang F. Antibacterial, cytotoxic activities and chemical composition of fruits of two Cameroonian *Zanthoxylum* species. Journal of Ethnopharmacology. 2013;**148**:74-80

[38] Mukhija M, Lal Dhar K, Nath Kalia A. Bioactive Lignans from *Zanthoxylum alatum* Roxb stem bark with cytotoxic potential. Journal of Ethnopharmacology. 2014;**152**:106-112

[39] Choumessi AT, Loureiro R, Silva AM, Moreira AC, Pieme AC, Tazoacha A, et al. Toxicity evaluation of some traditional African spices on breast cancer cells and isolated rat hepatic mitochondria. Food and Chemical Toxicology. 2012;**50**:4199-4208

[40] Mukhija M, Singh MP, Dhar KL, Kalia AN. Cytotoxic and antioxidant activity of *Zanthoxylum alatum* stem bark and its flavonoid constituents. Journal of Pharmacognosy and Phytochemistry. 2015;**4**:86-92

[41] Singh T, Meitei H, Sharma A, Robinson A, Singh L, Singh T. Anticancer properties and enhancement of therapeutic potential of cisplatin by leaf extract of *Zanthoxylum armatum* DC. Biological Research. 2015;**48**:46-55

[42] Karmakar I, Haldar S, Chakraborty M, Dewanjee S, Haldar PK. Antioxidant and cytotoxic activity of different extracts of *Zanthoxylum alatum*. Free Radicals and Antioxidants. 2015;**5**:21-28

[43] Karmakar I, Haldar S, Chakraborty M, Chaudhury K, Dewanjee S, Haldar PK. Regulation of apoptosis through bcl-2/bax proteins expression and DNA damage by *Zanthoxylum alatum*. Pharmaceutical Biology. 2016a;**54**:503-508

[44] Karmakar I, Haldar S, Chakraborty M, Dewanjee S, Haldar PK. *In vitro* antioxidant and cytotoxic activity of Zanthonitrile isolated from *Zanthoxylum alatum*. Journal of Applied Pharmaceutical Science. 2016b;**6**:119-122

[45] Nozaki R, Kono T, Bochimoto H, Watanabe T, Oketani K, Sakamaki Y, et al. *Zanthoxylum* fruit extract from Japanese pepper promotes autophagic cell death in cancer cells. Oncotarget. 2016;**7**:70437-70446

[46] Alam F, Saqib QN. Evaluation of *Zanthoxylum armatum* Roxb for *in vitro* biological activities. Journal of Traditional and Complementary Medicine. 2017;**7**:515-518

[47] Guetchueng ST, Nahar L, Ritchie KJ, Ismail FMD, Evans AR, Sarker SD. Zanthoamides G-I: Three

new alkamides from *Zanthoxylum zanthoxyloides*. Phytochemistry Letters. 2018;**26**:125-129

[48] Pang W, Liu S, He F, Li X, Saira B, Zheng T, et al. Anticancer activities of *Zanthoxylum bungeanum* seed oil on malignant melanoma. Journal of Ethnopharmacology. 2018;**229**:180-189

[49] Satria D, Silalahi J, Haro G, Ilyas S, Hasibuan PAZ. Chemical analysis and cytotoxic activity of N-hexane fraction of *Zanthoxylum acanthopodium* DC fruits. Rasayan Journal of Chemistry. 2019;**12**:803-808

[50] Satria D, Silalahi J, Haro G, Ilyas S, Hasibuan PAZ. Cell cycle inhibition of ethylacetate fraction of *Zanthoxylum acanthopodium* DC fruit against T47D cells. Open Access Macedonian Journal of Medical Sciences. 2019;**7**:726-729

[51] Nakamura T, Komai N, Isogami I, Ueno K, Ikegami F, One K. Memory and learning-enhancing effect of Daikenchuto, a traditional Japanese herbal medicine, in mice. Journal of Natural Medicines. 2006;**60**:64-67

[52] Chen SF, Li LF, Chen J, Wang XT, Huang HJ. The antidepressant effect of procyanidins extract from *Zanthoxylum bungeanum* maxim. On ovariectomized model mice. Journal of Wenzhou Medical University. 2015;**45**:260-264

[53] Tian JM, Wang Y, Xu YZ, Yu ZC, Wei AZ, Zhang WM, et al. Characterization of isobutyl hydroxyamides with NGF-potentiating activity from *Zanthoxylum bungeanum*. Bioorganic & Medicinal Chemistry Letters. 2016;**26**:338-342

[54] Mehta DK, Das R, Bhandari A. *In vitro* anthelmintic activity of seeds of *Zanthoxylum armatum* DC. Against *Pheretima posthuma*. International Journal of Green Pharmacy. 2012;**6**:26-28

[55] Goodman CD, Austarheim I, Mollard V, Mikolo B, Malterud KE, McFadden GI, et al. Natural products from *Zanthoxylum heitzii* with potent activity against the malaria parasite. Malaria Journal. 2016;**15**:1-8

[56] Pavela R, Govindarajan M. The essential oil from *Zanthoxylum monophyllum* a potential mosquito larvicide with low toxicity to the non-target fish *Gambusia affinis*. Journal of Pest Science. 2017;**90**:369-378

[57] Costa RS, Souza Filho OP, Junior OCSD, Silva JJ, Le Hyaric M, Santos MAV, et al. *In vitro* anti-leishmanial and antitrypanosomal activity of compounds isolated from the roots of *Zanthoxylum tingoassuiba*. Brazilian Journal of Pharmacognosy. 2018;**28**:551-558

[58] Guleria S, Kumar A. Antifungal activity of some Himalayan medicinal plants using direct bioautography. Journal of Cell and Molecular Biology. 2006;**5**:95-98

[59] Kamdem SSL, Belletti N, Tchoumbougnang F, Essia-Ngang JJ, Montanari C, Tabanelli G, et al. Effect of mild heat treatments on the antimicrobial activity of essential oils of *Curcuma longa*, *Xylopia aethiopica*, *Zanthoxylum xanthoxyloides* and *Zanthoxylum leprieurii* against *Salmonella enteritidis*. Journal of Essential Oil Research. 2015;**27**:52-60

[60] Cabral V, Luo X, Junqueira E, Costa SS, Mulhovo S, Duarte A, et al. Enhancing activity of antibiotics against *Staphylococcus aureus*: *Zanthoxylum capense* constituents and derivatives. Phytomedicine. 2015;**22**:469-476

[61] Chen X, Wang W, Wang C, Liu Z, Sun Q, Wang D. Quality evaluation and chemometric discrimination of *Zanthoxylum bungeanum* maxim leaves based on flavonoids profiles, bioactivity and HPLC-fingerprint in a common garden experiment. Industrial Crops and Products. 2019;**134**:225-233

[62] Mirza A, Kareem A, Nami S, Rehman S, Bhat S, Nishat N, et al. Copper oxide nanomaterials derived from *Zanthoxylum armatum* DC and *Berberis lycium* Royle plant species: Characterization, assessment of free radical scavenging and antibacterial activity. Chemistry & Biodiversity. 2019;**16**:e1900145

[63] Bunalema L, Fotso GW, Waako P, Tabuti J, Yeboah SO. Potential of *Zanthoxylum leprieurii* as a source of active compounds against drug resistant *Mycobacterium tuberculosis*. BMC Complementary and Alternative Medicine. 2017;**17**:4-9

[64] Batool F, Sabir SM, Rocha JBT, Shah AH, Saify ZS, Ahmed SD. Evaluation of antioxidant and free radical scavenging activities of fruit extract from *Zanthoxylum alatum*: A commonly used spice from Pakistan. Pakistan Journal of Botany. 2010;**42**:4299-4311

[65] Singh G, Kapoor IPS, Singh P, Heluani C, Lampasona M, Catalan CAN. Chemistry and antioxidant properties of essential oil and oleoresins extracted from the seeds of Tomer (*Zanthoxylum armatum* DC.). International Journal of Food Properties. 2013;**16**:288-300

[66] Zhang YJ, Wang DM, Yang LN, Zhou D, Zhang JF. Purification and characterization of flavonoids from the leaves of *Zanthoxylum bungeanum* and correlation between their structure and antioxidant activity. PLoS One. 2014;**9**:e105725

[67] Nooreen Z, Kumar A, Bawankule DU, Tandon S, Ali M, Xuan TD, et al. New chemical constituents from the fruits of *Zanthoxylum armatum* and its in vitro anti-inflammatory profile. Natural Product Research. 2019;**33**:665-672

[68] Liu X, Xu L, Liu L, Wang Y, Zhao Y, Kang Q, et al. Combination of essential oil from *Zanthoxylum bungeanum* maxim. And a microemulsion system: Permeation enhancement effect on drugs with different lipophilicity and its mechanism. Journal of Drug Delivery Science and Technology. 2019;**55**:101309

[69] Kaur V, Kumar T, Bora SK. Pharmacological evaluation of *Zanthoxylum armatum* root extract on analgesic and anti-inflammatory activity. Journal of Pharmacy Research. 2011;**4**:2561-2562

[70] He W, Puyvelde LV, Kimpe ND, Verbruggen L, Anthonissen K, Flaas MVD, et al. Chemical constituents and biological activities of *Zanthoxylum usambarense*. Phototherapy Research. 2002;**16**:66-70

[71] Nguyen PH, Zhao BT, Kim O, Le JH, Choi JS, Min BS, et al. Anti-inflammatory terpenylated coumarins from the leaves of *Zanthoxylum schinifolium* with α-glucosidase inhibitory activity. Journal of Natural Medicines. 2016;**70**:276-281

[72] Nooreen Z, Singh S, Singh DK, Tandon S, Ahmad A, Luqman S. Characterization and evaluation of bioactive polyphenolic constituents from *Zanthoxylum armatum* DC., a traditionally used plant. Biomedicine and Pharmacotherapy. 2017;**89**:366-375

[73] Karki H, Upadhayay K, Pal H, Singh R. Antidiabetic potential of *Zanthoxylum armatum* bark extract on streptozotocin-induced diabetic rats. International Journal of Green Pharmacy. 2014;**8**:77-83

[74] Kimani CN, Mbaria JM, Suleiman M, Gakuya D, Kiama SG. Antihyperglycemic activity of *Zanthoxylum chalybeum* stem bark extract in diabetic rats. Journal of Pharmacognosy. 2015;**4**:183-189

[75] Rynjah CV, Devi NN, Khongthaw N, Syiem D, Majaw S. Evaluation of the antidiabetic property of aqueous leaves

extract of *Zanthoxylum armatum* DC. Using *in vivo* and *in vitro* approaches. Journal of Traditional and Complementary Medicine. 2018;**8**:134-140

[76] Hieu TT, Kim S, Kwon HW, Ahn Y. Enhanced repellency of binary mixture of *Zanthoxylum piperitium* pericrap steam distillate or *Zanthoxylum armatum* seed oil constituents and *Calophyllum inophyllum* nut oil and their aerosols to *Stomyxs calcitrans*. Pest Management Science. 2010;**66**:1191-1198

[77] Hieu TT, Jung J, Kim S, Ahn Y, Kwon HW. Behavioural and electroantennogram response of the stable fly (*Stomoxys calcitrans* L.) to plant essential oils and their mixtures with attractants. Pest Management Science. 2014;**70**:163-172

[78] Hieu TT, Kim S, Ahn Y. Toxicity of *Zanthoxylum piperitum* and *Zanthoxylum armatum* oil constituents and related compounds to *Stomoxys calcitrans*. Journal of Medical Entomology. 2012;**49**:1084-1091

[79] Ross SA, Al-Azeib MA, Krishnavei KS, Fronczek FR, Burandt CL. Alkamides from the leaves of *Zanthoxylum syncarpum*. Journal of Natural Products. 2005;**68**:1297-1299

[80] Christofoli M, Costa ECC, Bicalho KU, de Cassia DV, Peixoto MF, Alves CCF, et al. Insecticidal effect of nanoencapsulated essential oils from *Zanthoxylum rhoifolium* (Rutaceae) in Bemisia tabaci populations. Industrial Crops and Products. 2015;**70**:301-308

[81] Wang C, You C, Yang K, Guo S, Geng Z, Fan L, et al. Antifeedant activities of methanol extracts of four *Zanthoxylum* species and benzophenanthridines from stem bark of *Zanthoxylum schinifolium* against *Tribolium castaneum*. Industrial Crops and Products. 2015b;**74**:407-411

[82] Wang C, Zhang W, You C, Guo S, Geng Z, Fan L, et al. Insecticidal constituents of essential oil derived from *Zanthoxylum armatum* against two stored product insects. Journal of Oleo Science. 2015a;**64**:861-868

[83] Kumar V, Reddy SGE, Chauhan U, Kumar N, Singh B. Chemical composition and larvicidal activity of *Zanthoxylum armatum* against diamondback moth *Plutella xylostella*. Natural Product Research. 2016;**30**:689-692

[84] Costa ECC, Christofoli M, de Costa GCS, Peixoto MF, Fernandes JB, Forim MR, et al. Essential oil repellent action of plants of the genus *Zanthoxylum* against *Bemisia tabaci* biotype B. (Homoptera: Aleyrodidae). Scientia Horticulturae. 2017;**226**:327-332

[85] Kim J, Seo S, Park K. Nematicidal activity of plant essential oil and components from *Gaultheria fragrantissima* and *Zanthoxylum alatum* against the pine wood nematode, *Bursaphelenchus xylophilus*. Nematology. 2011;**13**:87-93

[86] Kayani MZ, Mukhtar T, Hussain MA. Evaluation of nematicidal effects of *Cannabis sativa* L. and *Zanthoxylum alatum* Roxb. Against root-knot nematodes, Meloidogyne incognita. Crop Protection. 2012;**39**:52-56

[87] Lee SJ, Lim KT. Glycoprotein of *Zanthoxylum piperitum* DC has a hepatoprotective effect via anti-oxidative character *in vivo* and *in vitro*. Toxicology In Vitro. 2008;**22**:376-385

[88] Ranawat LS, Patel J. Antioxidant and hepatoprotective activity of ethanolic extracts of bark of Zanthoxylum armatum DC in paracetamol-induced hepatotoxicity. International Journal of Pharmaceutical Sciences and Drug Research. 2013;**5**:120-124

[89] Talluri MR, Gummadi VP, Battu GR, Killari KN. Evaluation of Hepatoprotective activity of *Zanthoxylum armatum* on paracetamol-induced liver toxicity in rats. Indian Journal of Pharmaceutical Sciences. 2018;**81**:138-145

[90] Zhang Z, Liu J, Shen P, Cao Y, Lu X, Gao X, et al. *Zanthoxylum bungeanum* pericarp extract prevents dextran sulfate sodium-induced experimental colitis in mice via the regulation of TLR4 and TLR4-related signaling pathways. International Immunopharmacology. 2016;**41**:127-135

[91] Heng L, Li C, Jia M, Yao XJ, Mei QB. Study on therapeutic effects of seed soil of *Zanthoxylum bungeanum* maxim. On experimental hyperlipidemia in rat. Chinese Medical Journal. 2005;**30**:1012-1013

[92] Mangalanathan M, Devendhiran T, Uthamaramasamy S, Kumarasamy K, Mohanraj K, Devendhiran K, et al. Efficacy of *Zanthoxylum armatum* fruit on isoproterenol induced myocardial infarction in rats. South Asian Journal of Engineering and Technology. 2019;**8**:4-11

[93] Jiang L, Kubota K. Formation by mechanical stimulus of the flavor compounds in young leaves of Japanese pepper (*Xanthoxylum piperitum* DC). Journal of Agricultural and Food Chemistry. 2001;**49**:1353-1357

[94] Ji Y, Li S, Ho C. Chemical composition, sensory properties and application of Sichuan pepper (*Zanthoxylum* genus). Food Science and Human Wellness. 2019;**8**:115-125

[95] Wu G, Wu H. Analgesia synergism of essential oil from pericarp of *Zanthoxylum schinifolium* and verapamil. Evidence-based Complementary and Alternative Medicine. 2014;**2014**:505876

[96] Oh M, Chung MS. Effects of oils and essential oils from seeds of *Zanthoxylum schinifolium* against foodborne viral surrogates. Evidence-Based Complementary and Alternative Medicine. 2014;**2014**:1-6

[97] Ravindran PN, Divakaran M, Pillai GS. Other herbs and spices: Achiote to Szechuan pepper. In: Handbook of Herbs and Spices. Vol. 2. Cambridge, United Kingdom: Woodhead Publishing Series in Food Science, Technology and Nutrition; 2012. pp. 534-556

[98] Zhu RX, Zhong K, Zeng WC, He XY, Gu XQ, Zhao ZF, et al. Essential oil composition and antibacterial activity of *Zanthoxylum bungeanum*. African Journal of Microbiology Research. 2011;**5**:4631-4637

[99] Sugai E, Morimitsu Y, Kubota K. Quantitative analysis of sanshool compounds in Japanese pepper (*Xanthoxylum piperitum* DC.) and their pungent characteristics. Bioscience, Biotechnology, and Biochemistry. 2005a;**69**:1958-1962

[100] Sugai E, Morimitsu Y, Iwasaki Y, Morita A, Watanabe T, Kubota K. Pungent qualities of sanshool-related compounds evaluated by a sensory test and activation of rat TRPV1. Bioscience, Biotechnology, and Biochemistry. 2005b;**69**:1951-1957

[101] Zeng M, Wang J, Zhang M, Chen J, He Z, Qin F, et al. Inhibitory effects of Sichuan pepper (*Zanthoxylum bungeanum*) and sanshoamide extract on heterocyclic amine formation in grilled ground beef patties. Food Chemistry. 2018;**239**:111-118

Chapter 6

Metabolomics

Naveen Kumar Dubey

Abstract

The aim of this chapter is to make a brief understanding on Metabolomics identification, extraction, and analysis techniques. As the name suggests, Metabolomics is the study of metabolites present in the body fluid (blood, plasma, urine, and saliva) or body parts (muscles, bone, tissue, and cells). These might be known metabolites or unknown metabolites. The metabolites can be endogenous (present in the body) or exogenous (formed by consuming external medicinal product). The molecular mass of these metabolites is usually lower (50–1500 Dalton) than the proteins and macromolecules. These metabolites can be extracted using various techniques such as solid phase extraction, liquid-liquid extraction, or simple protein precipitation. Extracted sample of metabolite then can be analyzed qualitatively or quantitatively using numerous analytical techniques such as high performance liquid chromatography (HPLC), liquid chromatography mass spectrometry (LC–MS/MS), dry blood spot (DBS), infrared (IR) spectroscopy, ultraviolet visible (UV) spectroscopy, nuclear magnetic resonance (NMR), ELISA, and chemiluminescence. Sensitivity of detection is the key factor, among many others, to decide which technique would be suitable for analysis. Liquid chromatography mass spectrometry (LC–MS/MS) is the latest and most sensitive technique among all the available methodology till date that has been extensively and exclusively used in current scenario.

Keywords: known metabolite, unknown metabolite, extraction, LC–MS/MS analysis, HPLC analysis, NMR analysis

1. Introduction

Current development, demand, and innovation in the field of science have made a tremendous effort to reduce the load of chemical/biologics in human body from gram to microgram level. Now scientists are evaluating how harmful is the effect of these chemicals (drugs) when consumed by any route in human body. Recent FDA/other regulatory agency examples are the presence of five to seven nitrosamine impurities (metabolites) (e.g., NDMA family) in sartan (e.g., valsartan, telmisartan, etc.) or ranitidine [1]. Lower therapeutic dose would be one of the solutions to reduce the level of these metabolites to an acceptable level in human matrix.

The metabolome is a close counterpart to the genome, the transcriptome, and the proteome. Together these four 'omes' constitute the building blocks of systems biology. Metabolomics is a newly emerging field of research concerned with the high-throughput identification and quantification of the small molecule metabolites in the metabolome. The metabolome can be defined as the complete complement of all small molecule (<1500 Da) metabolites found in a specific cell, organ, or organism. Metabolites are small molecules that are chemically transformed during metabolism and can provide a functional readout of the

IntechOpen

cellular state. Metabolites, unlike genes and proteins, serve as direct signatures of biochemical activity and are much easier to correlate with phenotype. One of the challenges of systems biology and functional genomics is to integrate proteomic, transcriptomic, and metabolomic information to give a more complete picture of living organisms. While mRNA gene expression data and proteomic analyses do not tell the whole story of what might be happening in a cell, metabolic profiling can give an instantaneous snapshot of the physiology of that cell [2–6]. Pictorial diagram of all the omics interrelated to each other has been shown in **Figures 1** and **2**.

The metabolites formed in the body can be generated either by Phase 1 or Phase 2 metabolic pathway [7]. The representation of these pathways is shown in **Figure 3**.

Regulatory guidance and agencies are emphasizing on the need of identification and analysis of each possible molecule separately and in combination with the intended matrix to generalize the pros and cons of that particular drug before human use [8–11].

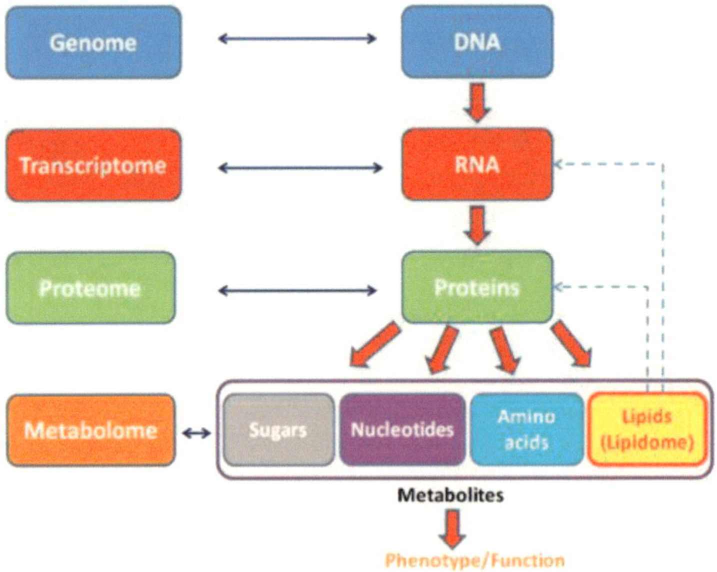

Figure 1.
The "omics" cascade.

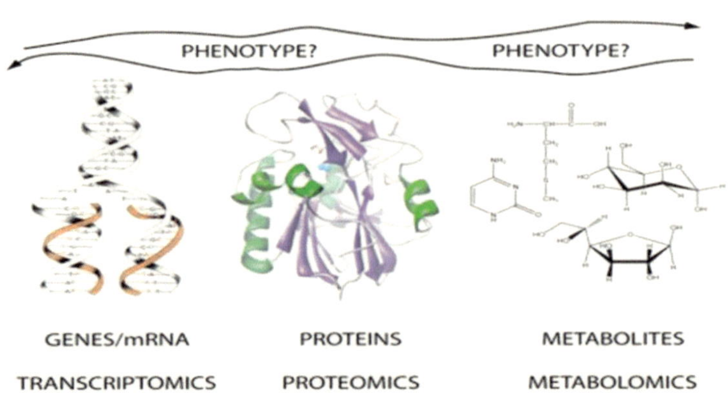

Figure 2.
Genes to phenotype.

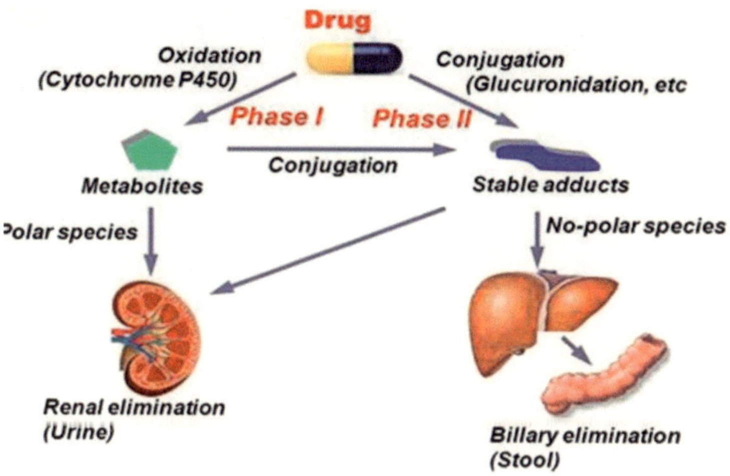

Figure 3.
Metabolite pathways in human.

2. Metabolite extraction technique

When it comes to extract the metabolites from the bio-fluid (blood, plasma, serum, saliva, or urine), mainly three methodologies are prevailing. These are as follows.

2.1 Protein precipitation

This technique is very useful for high throughput as it involves only centrifugation step when a precipitating agent is added to matrix (plasma, blood, or serum). The basic principle for this technique is the amount or volume of precipitating agent must be sufficient to precipitate the protein present in the matrix. Selection of precipitating agent also depends on the technique involved for analysis of the compound of interest. For example, trichloroacetic acid (TCA), perchloric acid (PCA), and zinc sulfate ($ZnSO_4$) are not suitable for mass spectrometer (MS) analysis, whereas these are suitable for high performance liquid chromatography (HPLC) analysis [12]. Organic solvents such as methanol or acetonitrile are suitable for both HPLC and LC–MS/MS analysis [13–15]. The amount of precipitating agent varies for precipitating the matrix. TCA or PCA can be used directly (20–50 μL) in 500 μL of matrix [16–19]. Organic solvent should be 2–3 times the volume of matrix. After centrifugation, either sample can be directly injected into the HPLC or LC–MS/MS or it can be concentrated in nitrogen evaporator followed by reconstitution. Centrifugation also plays an important role for this methodology [20]. Higher the revolution per minute (RPM) speed (~15,000 RPM) higher would be the sedimentation of particle and cleaner would be the sample. Flow of protein precipitation is shown in **Figure 4**.

The drawback of this technique is high matrix effect, low recovery if the compound of interest is associated with precipitated protein.

2.2 Liquid-Liquid extraction

The liquid-liquid extraction (LLE) technique [21–25] is one of the widely used methodologies to extract most of the metabolites from bio-matrix. The basic principle of this technique is portioning or separation of compound from one

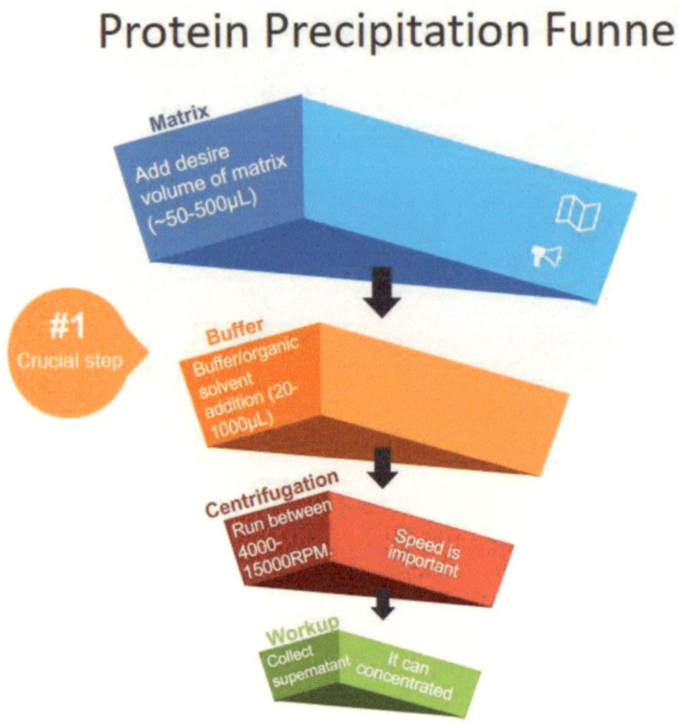

Figure 4.
Protein precipitation process.

liquid part to another one depending on its affinity. As we know, our body fluid (plasma ... urine) is polar in nature; hence, less polar or nonpolar solvents such as ether/t-butyl methyl ether/ethyl acetate/dichloromethane are used to extract the compounds from the human matrix. The LLE technique can be used in many ways such as manual or automatic. Manual methodology would be cost effective when intelligent approach like freeze flash (using dry ice and methanol) is used along with vortexing the sample at high speed (2000–2500 RPM). Typical sample volume versus solvent volume is required in 1:3 ratio for proper extraction. Solvent needs to be evaporated in a nitrogen evaporator under constant temperature and pressure. The dried sample should be reconstituted in an appropriate solution for analysis on either HPLC or LC–MS/MS. Typical flow of the process is shown in **Figure 5**.

2.3 Solid-phase extraction

The cleanest process in extraction methodology is solid-phase extraction (SPE). This process involves the adsorption of compound on the solid surface (bed) of a polymeric membrane with a covalent and ionic interaction. Desorption of molecule takes place when a strong solvent/solution is passed through the surface of cartridge. Umpteen of SPE cartridge is available in the market staring from C18 to ionic (cation or anion) with weak and strong combination [26–28]. The cartridge can be of different platform like well plate of tube type. The polymeric membrane may vary from few milligram to few gram depending on the requirement of analysis. Matrix as low as 50 µL to as high as 3 mL can be employed for extraction using different format of SPE platform. Different kinds of protocols are used to

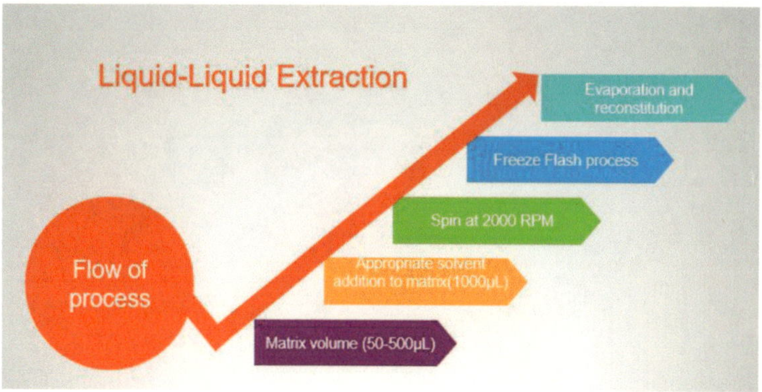

Figure 5
Liquid liquid extraction methodology.

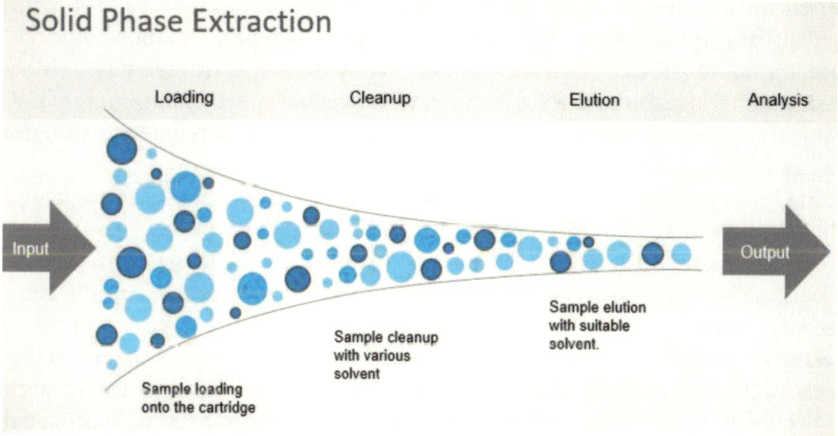

Figure 6.
Solid phase extraction technique.

clean up the sample from matrix, which depend on the various trials conducted during development stage. SPE unit can be operated in both negative pressure mode (using vacuum manifold) and positive pressure mode (using nitrogen gas). Clean sample can be either directly injected into the HPLC or LC–MSMS system or concentrated to get high recovery. Pictorial presentation on SPE process is shown in **Figure 6**.

3. Dry blood spot technique

When there is a challenge of low sample volume (e.g., neonatal), it is advisable to look for innovation in this area. Dry blood spot (DBS) is a very useful technique that can support the low volume sample analysis. Just a spot is required on the polymeric membrane that can be cut in a circular shape using specific tools. The cut part then can be dissolved in a suitable solvent and directly injected on the high sensitive instrument for analysis [29–31]. The major challenge for this method is sensitivity achievement on the analytical instrument. Mass spectrometers (latest models) are the only way out for such kind of analysis (**Figure 7**).

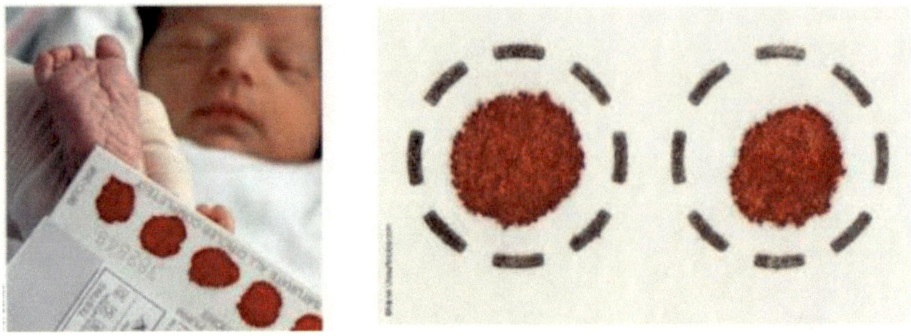

Figure 7.
Dry blood spot technique.

4. Metabolite analysis technique

There are a variety of analytical techniques that could be employed for metabolites identification and its analysis. Few of them are high performance liquid chromatography (HPLC), liquid chromatography mass spectrometry (LC–MSMS), nuclear magnetic resonance (NMR), ultraviolet visible spectrophotometer (UV), and infrared spectrophotometer (IR). Among all these, most reliable techniques are HPLC and LC–MSMS.

HPLC is a good technique for the analysis of formulation product in aqueous medium (nonhuman matrix) as there is no limitation of sample volume, concentration, and its detection. However, it would be a challenge when the analysis is to be done in human matrix due to obvious reason of low sample volume and hence its sensitivity on the instrument. Sensitivity on HPLC can be enhanced by replacing the UV detector by RF (fluorescence) detector provided the molecule if fluorescence is active. Derivatization methodology can also enhance the sensitivity of molecule by adding some auxochromes or chromophores to the main molecule moiety. Few examples are presented in **Table 1**, where parent molecules are not sensitive enough as such on HPLC analysis, however, using derivatizing reagent, sensitivity got enhanced.

Liquid chromatography when connected with mass spectrometer as detector, sensitivity of the molecule enhanced many folds by virtue of mass to charge (m/z) ratio detection. By enlarge, mass spectrometer is the only technique in the field of biomolecules and its analysis, by which one can quantitate the metabolites up to pg/ml level.

In the mass spectrometer, ion source plays a crucial role to ionize the molecule of interest. Basically, there are two kinds of ion sources predominantly used in

S. No	Molecule has low sensitivity (on HPLC)	Derivatizing agent	Complex has high sensitivity (on HPLC)
1	Ethinyl estradiol	Dansyl chloride	Ethinyl estradiol-Dansyl complex
2	Valproic acid	2-bromo-2′-acetonaphthone	Valproic-acid-2-bromo-2′-acetonaphthone complex
3	Alendronate	Diazomethane	Alendronate-Diazomethane complex
4	Mesalamine	Acetic anhydride	Mesalamine-Acetic anhydride complex

Table 1.
Molecule with derivatizing reagent.

entire pharma industry or academics. These are Electron spray ionization (ESI) and Atmospheric pressure chemical ionization (APCI).

4.1 Electro spray ionization (ESI)

The molecules of interest are first introduced into the ionization source of the mass spectrometer using an HPLC (or UPLC) system, where they are first ionized to acquire positive or negative charges. The liquid associated with molecules get evaporated due to high temperature. Thereafter, due to coulombic repulsion between the ion, charged particles are formed. The ions then travel through the mass analyzer and arrive at different parts of the detector according to their mass/charge (m/z) ratio. After the ions make contact with the detector, usable signals are generated and recorded by a computer system. The computer displays the signals graphically as a mass spectrum showing the relative abundance of the signals according to their m/z ratio. A typical pictorial diagram is shown in **Figure 8**.

4.2 Atmospheric pressure chemical ionization (APCI)

The APCI source is selected for molecules, which are thermally stable as the basic principle works on the fact of charge transfer from solvent molecule to the compound of interest in the ion source using corona discharge tube. The other operation in this ion source would remain same as ESI like transfer of ions from ion source to vacuum region and selective monitoring up to detector. APCI diagram is shown in **Figure 9**.

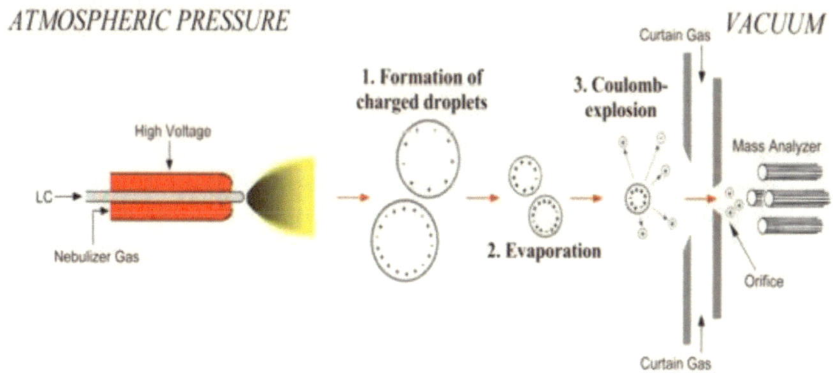

Figure 8.
Electro spray ionisation mechanism.

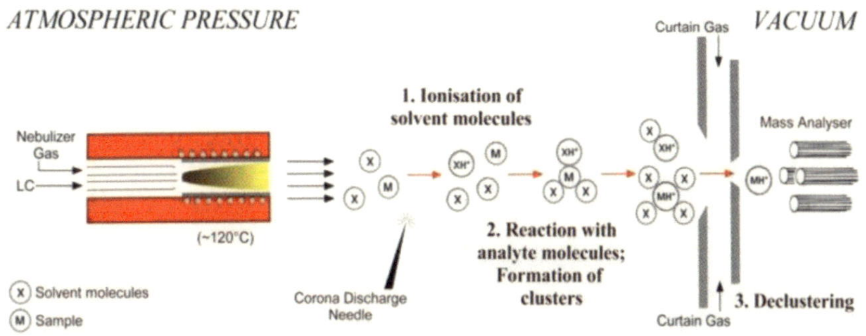

Figure 9.
Atmospheric pressure chemical ionisation mechanism.

S. No	Parameter	HPLC	LC–MS/MS
1	Run time	High (5–100 min)	Low (2–10 min)
2	Ratio of mobile phase	High aqueous (~70%) with low organic solvent (~30%)	Low aqueous (~30%) with high organic solvent (~70%)
3	Column	15–30 cm	5–15 cm
4	Efficiency	Low	High
5	Sensitivity	Low	High
6	Feasibility of analysis	Low	High
7	Injection volume	Low	High
8	Matrix volume	Low	High
9	Cost	Low	High

Table 2.
Comparison between HPLC and LC–MS/MS.

Both HPLC and LC-MS/MS techniques can be employed for identification and quantitation of metabolites in human matrix; however, both have some limitation and benefits. **Table 2** represents the basic difference between both the techniques:

5. Conclusions

Metabolites are the compounds generated by our body after the consumption of drug substance. Some of these metabolites are known, and most of them are unknown. They may be harmful, beneficial, or inactive in the body. Extraction and detection are thus very important to understand complete behavior of these metabolites. Sensitive analytical technique like LC–MS/MS is the most employed methodology by most of the pharmaceutical/diagnostic companies as one can detect parent and all possible metabolites in one single run within 10- to 50-min time in human matrix.

Acknowledgements

The author acknowledges the support of his professor B.I Fozdar for constant guidance and his family (Wife, Aradhna & Son, Arnav) for standing by him all the time.

Conflict of interest

There is no conflict of interest on publishing of this chapter.

Notes/Thanks/Other declarations

The author is thankful to all his team mates for supporting to write this chapter.

DOI: http://dx.doi.org/10.5772/intechopen.92423

Author details

Naveen Kumar Dubey
Indira Gandhi National Open University, New Delhi, India

*Address all correspondence to: nd005@rediffmail.com

References

[1] FDA Updates and Press Announcements on Angiotensin II Receptor Blocker (ARB) Recalls (Valsartan, Losartan, and Irbesartan). Available from: https://www.fda.gov/drugs/drug-safety-and-availability/fda-updates-and-press-announcements-angiotensin-ii-receptor-blocker-arb-recalls-valsartan-losartan

[2] Oliver SG, Winson MK, Kell DB, Baganz F. Systematic functional analysis of the yeast genome. Trends in Biotechnology. 1998;**16**:373-378

[3] Yadav SP. The wholeness in suffix -omics, -omes, and the word om. Journal of Biomolecular Techniques. 2007;**18**:277

[4] Wanjek C. Systems biology as defined by NIH. NIH Catalyst. Available from: https://irp.nih.gov/catalyst/v19i6/systems-biology-as-defined-by-nih

[5] Dettmer K, Aronov PA, Hammock BD. Mass spectrometry-based metabolomics. Mass Spectrometry Reviews. 2007;**26**:51-78

[6] Patti GJ, Yanes O, Siuzdak G. Innovation: Metabolomics: The apogee of the omics trilogy. Nature Reviews. Molecular Cell Biology. 2012;**13**:263-269

[7] Phase-I vs. Phase II Metabolism. Available from: https://step1.medbullets.com/pharmacology/107006/phase-i-vs-phase-ii-metabolism

[8] Bioanalytical Method Validation Guidance for Industry. 2018. Available from: https://www.fda.gov/downloads/drugs/guidances/ucm070107.pdf

[9] Dubey NK, Fozdar BI. Interconversion from N-Desmethyl clomipramine to clomipramine and its impact on a bioequivalence study. Separation Science Plus. 2018;**1**:714-725

[10] Guideline on Bioanalytical Method Validation [Online]. 2012. Available from: http://www.ema.europa.eu/docs/en_GB/document_library/Scientific_guideline/2011/08/WC500109686.pdf

[11] Overcoming the Charged Ion Competition in Triple Quad Chemical Ionization Ion Source for Estimation of Celecoxib in Biological Matrix and its Application to Bioequivalence Study. Drug Res/2019-03-1789/7.8.2019/MPS

[12] Di L, Kerns EH. Profiling drug-like properties in discovery research. Current Opinion in Chemical Biology. 2003;**7**(3):402-408

[13] White RE. High-throughput screening in drug metabolism and pharmacokinetic support in drug discovery. Annual Review of Pharmacology and Toxicology. 2000;**40**:133-157

[14] Ulrich R, Friend SH. Toxicogenomics and drug discovery: Will new technologies help us produce better drugs? Nature reviews. Drug Discovery. 2002;**1**:84-88

[15] Tarbit MH, Berman J. High-throughput approaches for evaluating absorption, distribution, metabolism and excretion properties of lead compounds. Current Opinion in Chemical Biology. 1998;**2**(3):411-416

[16] Masimirembwa CM, Thompson R, Andersson TB. Handbook of pharmaceutical analysis. Combinatorial Chemistry & High Throughput Screening. 2001;**4**(3):245-263

[17] Dean JH, Olson HM. The integration of investigative toxicology in the drug discovery process. Biology of the Cell. 1993;**77**(1):3-8

[18] Atterwill CK, Wing MG. In vitro preclinical lead optimisation

technologies (PLOTs) in pharmaceutical development. Toxicology Letters. 2002;**127**(1-3):143-151

[19] Amidon GL, Lennernas H, Shah VP, Crison JR. A theoretical basis for a biopharmaceutic drug classification: the correlation of in vitro drug product dissolution and in vivo bioavailability. Pharmaceutical Research. 1995;**12**(3):413-420

[20] Meugge I. Selection criteria for drug-like compounds. Medicinal Research Reviews. 2003;**23**(3):302-321

[21] Fardy JJ, Ishimori T, Navratil JD, Sato T, Schulz WW. Solvent extraction applied to nuclear science. Atomic Energy Review. Available from: https://inis.iaea.org/collection/NCLCollectionStore/_Public/14/777/14777334.pdf

[22] Rice NM. Recommended nomenclature for solvent extraction. Chemistry & Industry. 1977;**3**(6):718-723

[23] Misek T, editor. Recommended Systems for Liquid Extraction Studies. London: Institute of Chemical Engineers; 1978

[24] Roddy JW, McDowell WJ. Separation Systems Data Base: A Users' Manual, Revision 1. Oak Ridge National Laboratory operated by Union Carbide Corporation for the USA department of Energy. ORNL/TM-6593/R1. 1978

[25] Wisniak J, Tamir A. Liquid–Liquid Equilibrium and Extraction. Amsterdam: Elsevier; 1980

[26] Kinsella B, O'Mahony J, Malone E, et al. Current trends in sample preparation for growth promoter and veterinary drug residue analysis. Journal of Chromatography A. 2009;**1216**(46):7977-8015

[27] Wen Y, Zhang M, Zhao Q, Feng Y-Q. Monitoring of five sulfonamide antibacterial residues in milk by in-tube solid-phase microextraction coupled to high-performance liquid chromatography. Journal of Agricultural and Food Chemistry. 2005;**53**(22):8468-8473

[28] Barlow J. Antimicrobial resistance and the use of antibiotics in the dairy industry: Facing consumer perceptions and producer realities. Advances in Dairy Technology;**23**:47-58

[29] World Health Organization. Cardiovascular Diseases (CVDs). 2017. Available from: http://www.who.int/mediacentre/factsheets/fs317/en/

[30] Lawes CM, Hoorn SV, Rodgers A. Global burden of blood-pressure-related disease, 2001. The Lancet. 2008;**371**(9623):1513-1518

[31] Campbell DJ, Mcgrady M, Prior DL, et al. Most individuals with treated blood pressures above target receive only one or two antihypertensive drug classes. Internal Medicine Journal. 2013;**43**(2):137-143

Chapter 7

The Antibacterial Activity of *Mentha*

Monique Mancuso

Abstract

The topic of this chapter is the antibacterial activity of *Mentha* against several pathogenic bacteria. Some aromatic plants are recently being studied for their antibacterial properties, such as citrus essential oils, *Armoracia rusticana*, etc., showing inhibition against bacteria, fungi and yeasts. This chapter highlights the antibacterial characteristics of *Mentha piperita* (peppermint) and other *Mentha* sp. that are used daily as folk remedies and in food industry too. *Mentha* acts as counterirritant and analgesic with the ability to reduce pain and improve blood flow to the affected area. For these reasons, mint essential oils are well studied due to their antibacterial activities against both Gram-negative and Gram-positive ones and can be useful as a substitute to some antibiotics and combat the antimicrobial bacterial resistance.

Keywords: *Mentha* sp., antibacterial activity, plants, leaf extract, essential oils

1. Introduction

The essential oils (EOs) are a group of several natural chemicals that are characterised by their volatility and aroma [1].

The essential oils are produced by different plant parts (flowers, buds, seeds, leaves, twigs, bark, herbs, wood, fruits and roots) as secondary metabolites [2]. The EOs are about 3000, 300 of which are used for pharmaceutical, agronomic, food, sanitary, cosmetic and perfusion purposes [2]. They are a complex of natural mixtures of lipophilic substances and consist of two fractions: volatile (from 85 to 99%) and non-volatile, the second one being a heavier fraction than the first one (from 1 to 15%) [3]. Hydrocarbon compounds and oxygenated compounds prevail in the volatile fraction of EOs. The oxygenated fraction gives the characteristic flavour to the essences, while terpenes and sesquiterpenes perform a support function. The separation process of terpenes, as well as improving the stability of the essence, allows to concentrate the oxygenate fraction that it brings a superior contribution to perfume and aroma. The non-volatile fraction consists of many classes of substances such as high molecular weight hydrocarbons, fatty acids, steroids, carotenoids, waxes, coumarins, psoralenes and flavonoids [2]. Several EOs extracted from plants contain compounds that are responsible for their antimicrobial effects [4–6]. The mechanisms by which different EOs are capable of damaging bacteria depend on their composition. Generally, antimicrobial activity is derived not only from a single mechanism of action but also from a cascade of reactions that involve the entire bacterial cell because EOs have several chemical structures in their composition and, consequently, several functional groups. In general, Gram-positive bacteria are more susceptible to the effects of EOs than Gram-negative

IntechOpen

bacteria, due to significant structural differences in the cell wall of these two groups of bacteria [7, 8]. The structure of Gram-positive bacteria facilitates the penetration of hydrophobic molecules into the cell and acts on the bacterial wall, cytoplasmic membrane or cytoplasm [1].

The diseases caused by bacterial pathogens are a great concern all over the world [9]. Since the beginning of the 1980s, it is observed that the number of antimicrobial agents decreased considerably, while the resistance of the microorganisms to them has been growing in a fast way due to the development of new resistance mechanisms [10].

For these reasons, nowadays, there has been a growing interest in the determination of the biological and antimicrobial properties of herb extracts derived from several medicinal plants [11]. Among the species of plants from which essential oils are obtained, there is mint (*Mentha* sp.), in fact, which is used all over the world as flavouring agent in cosmetics, in pharmaceutical products as well as food including candy and gum and for liqueur [12]. The genus *Mentha*, family Labiatae, consists of about 25 species. Native from the temperate areas of the world is common in Eurasia, North America, southern Africa, and Australia, mints are widely distributed throughout. Mint essential oil is produced by their leaves [13–20]. Mint essential oils (MEOs) are used as scents in perfumery. Some species are commonly used in herbal medicine. The antibacterial effects of mint species, in particular peppermint oil from *Mentha piperita*, spearmint oil from *Mentha spicata* var. *crispa* and corn mint oil from *Mentha arvensis,* have great antibacterial activity against *Staphylococcus aureus, Streptococcus pyogenes* and *B. subtilis* [1, 9, 21]. *Mentha pulegium* showed activity against *S. aureus* and *Enterococcus faecalis* [11].

Mentha spicata and other *Mentha* species showed activity against Gram-negative bacteria; the former is active against biofilm cultures of *Vibrio* spp. [22]; *Mentha longifolia* is active against *Salmonella typhimurium* [23]; and *Mentha pulegium* inhibits the growth of *Pseudomonas sp., E. coli and Pseudomonas aeruginosa* [11, 24, 25].

2. Chemical composition of *Mentha* species essential oil

The essential oils from different *Mentha* species have been isolated by hydrodistillation using Clevenger apparatus or pharmacopoeia distillation apparatus [26].

The composition of MEOs that gives the characteristic peppermint aroma and flavour is menthol and pulegone [27], whereas for spearmint, it was reported that the flavour is due to carvone [28].

Several investigations have been carried out on the chemical composition of different samples of *Mentha* species from different geographical regions revealing that chemical composition and percentage varied depending upon the species and the harvesting time at different stages, and the geography as well as the extraction methods [29]. Some factors like physiological and environmental conditions, genetics and evolution also determine the chemical variability of *Mentha* essential oils [30]. Additionally, most of the species chemically characterised were rich in pulegone, menthone, menthol, carvone, 1,8-cineole, limonene and b-caryophyllene. For example, the chemical composition of the essential oil of *M. piperita* has abundant quantities of menthone, menthol and menthyl acetate, which varies based on different countries: in Serbia, menthone was 12.7%, menthol 37.4% and menthyl acetate 17.4% [31]. In Pakistan, the major components of *M. piperita* reported are menthone and menthol [32]. In India, menthol was (30–55%), menthofuran and menthyl acetate (1.0–9.2%) [33]. In Iran, *M. piperita EO* contains menthol (36.24%) and menthone (32.42%) as main constituents [34]. In Turkey, the reported chemical constituents of peppermint oil are menthone (44.1%), menthol (29.5%), menthyl-acetate (3.8%) and menthofuran (0.9%) [35]. However, in Korea, *M. piperita* leaves EO has different composition and include limonene (64.5 and 94.2%), 1,8-cineole (46.1%), p-menth-2-en-ol (34.5%), menthol (33.4%) and linalyl-acetate (28.2%) as main components [36]. These differences can influence the antibacterial capacity with respect to one pathogenic bacteria species; it is important to note that it is not a single compound but the combination of the chemical compounds that carries the specific antimicrobial activity [37, 38]. The hydrophobicity is one of the major distinctiveness of essential oils, which enables their assimilation into the cell membrane. The MEO oil rich in menthol and compounds similar to menthol shows that the hydroxyl group and the presence of a system of delocalized electrons are important for the antimicrobial activity. These similar compounds destabilise the cytoplasmic membrane and, also, act as a proton exchanger, thereby reducing the pH gradient across the cytoplasmic membrane. The resulting collapse of the proton motive force and depletion of the ATP pool eventually lead to cell death [39].

3. Methods for testing the antibacterial activity of essential oils

The methods used for testing antimicrobial activity of EOs are the disc diffusion method, the determination of minimum inhibitory concentration (MIC) and the vapour phase method. Another method is the use of TLC-bioautography.

3.1 Agar diffusion test

In the agar diffusion test, the EO to be tested is placed on the top of an agar surface. There are two techniques: in the first one, the essential oil is adsorbed onto a sterile paper disk; in the second one, the EO is put inside a hole into the agar surface. Then, the agar plates are incubated according to the physiological characteristics of the tested bacteria. The antimicrobial agent tested by spreading in the medium inhibits bacterial growth, thereby creating halos of inhibition around the bacterial colonies; the size of inhibition zone is regarded as a measure for the antimicrobial potency of an essential oil [40]. But some lipophilic compounds such as farnesol, although the compound results in a strong inhibition in the serial dilution test [41], cause only small inhibition zones, i.e. against *Bacillus subtilis* [42]. Thus, strong inhibitors having low water solubility gave a poor or even negative result in the agar diffusion test. For this reason, it is better to perform different tests. Similarly, it is important to interpret the size of inhibition zones, which depends on both the diffusion coefficient and antimicrobial activity of every compound present in an essential oil [43].

3.2 Dilution test

In the dilution test, the essential oil to be tested is incorporated in a semisolid agar medium or liquid broth in several defined amounts. The absence of growth in agar plates or test tubes is determined with the naked eye after incubation. The minimum inhibitory concentration (MIC) is the concentration of essential oil present in the ungrown agar plate or test tube with the highest amount of test material. When essential oils are tested, the main difficulty is caused by their low water solubility. The addition of solvents (e.g. dimethylsulfoxide and ethanol) or detergents (e.g. Tween 20) to the growth medium is unavoidable, which however influences the MIC [44–46]. Another problem is the volatilisation of essential oils during incubation. Furthermore, MIC-influencing test parameters are the size of inoculum, the pH of growth medium and the incubation time.

Nevertheless, the serial dilution test in liquid broth was recommended for natural substances [47] and is standardised for the testing of antibacterial and antifungal drugs in liquid broth and agar plates [48]. Its use enables a link to data of pharmaceutical drugs and an easier interpretation of test results. All concentrations are recalculated in μg/ml [1, 49].

3.3 Vapour phase test

The components of EOs and their relative volatilities determine the characteristics of their vapours, which in turn affect the antimicrobial potential [50, 51]. For this test, a standardised method for testing the antimicrobial activity of essential oils does not exist. Recently, several studies confirmed that vapour phases of EOs are more effective antimicrobials than their liquid phases [51–53] probably because the lipophilic molecules in the aqueous phase associate to form micelles and thus suppress the attachment of the EOs to the organism, whereas the vapour phase allows free attachment [54].

3.4 TLC bioautography

Direct bioautography combined with thin layer chromatographic (TLC) separation is a rapid and sensitive screening method for the detection of antimicrobial compounds. Test microorganism cultures are capable of growing directly on the TLC plate, so each step of the assay is performed on the sorbent. Similar to the common antimicrobial screening methods, TLC bioautography must be carried out under controlled conditions, since the experimental conditions (e.g. solvent, sample application, resolution of compounds, type of microorganism and incubation time) may influence the result [55]. The advantages of direct bioautography are that it is suitable for evaluating complex plant extracts and facilitates rapid, economic and easy evaluation. The use of bioautography to detect antimicrobial compounds effective against plant and human pathogenic bacteria has been reported in the literature [56, 57].

4. Uses of mint essential oils

The mint species has always been widely used; the leaves, flowers, and stems of *Mentha* spp. are used traditionally in herbal teas or in several folk remedies for treatment [58, 59]. Recently, mint essential oil, as well as other plant essential oils, can be used as food preservative, in fact, there is a growing interest in the development of edible and biodegradable films for food made from bio-polymers, conservation and preservation instead of the synthetic preservatives and chemical additives once, that can cause intoxication, cancer and other degenerative diseases [60]. In addition, biobased active packaging facilitates continuous migration of active components into the food remaining at high concentrations for a prolonged time period [61]. Mint essential oil contains phenolic compounds such as α-pinene, citronellol, and methyl eugenol, which have antimicrobial activity against a wide range of microorganisms and antioxidant activity; for these reasons, MEOs are widely used as food additives and in pharmaceutical industries because they are considered as potent film additives that help in preventing lipid oxidation and microbial spoilage of foods [62]. Another interesting idea was to add mint essential oil (MEO) into gelatin-based edible films with an effective inhibition of microbial growth on the film surface [63]. Moreover, MEOs are also used both in agriculture to fight bacterial and fungal diseases [64] and to give other examples and in aquaculture as an additive in fish feed to increase immune defences, but also as sedative and anaesthetic for farmed fish [65].

5. Conclusion

MEOs have antibacterial effects against a wide range of pathogenic microorganisms in humans, fish, and vegetables also. MEOs' antibacterial activity is linked to their chemical composition rich in pulegone, menthone, menthol, carvone, 1, 8-cineole, limonene and b-caryophyllene and phenolic compounds also such as α-pinene, citronellol and methyl eugenol. For these reasons, MEOs are widely used as food additives and in pharmaceutical industries to prevent microbial spoilage of foods. The most used methods to test the antimicrobial activity of EOs are the disc diffusion method, the determination of minimum inhibitory concentration (MIC), and the vapour phase method, and to have the most truthful analysis possible on the antibacterial characteristics, it is better to use more than one method. The use of MEOs, and in general of EOs, is very important because being natural substances and therefore easily biodegradable, it could be a promising alternative to synthetic materials to fight the increasingly common bacterial infections.

Conflict of interest

The author declares no conflict of interest.

Author details

Monique Mancuso[1,2]

1 Institute for Marine Biological Resources and Biotechnology (IRBIM), National Research Council (CNR), Section of Messina, Messina, Italy

2 Anton Dohrn Zoological Station (CIS-Italy), Italy

*Address all correspondence to: monique.mancuso@cnr.it

References

[1] Horváth P, Koščová J. *In vitro* antibacterial activity of *Mentha* essential oils against *Staphylococcus aureus*. Folia Veterinaria. 2017;**61**:71-77. DOI: 10.1515/fv-2017-0030

[2] Palazzolo E, Laudicina VA, Germanà MA. Current and potential use of citrus essential oils. Current Organic Chemistry. 2013;**17**:3042-3049

[3] Dugo P, Ragonese C, Russo M, Sciarrone D, Santi L, Cotroneo A, et al. Sicilian lemon oil: Composition of volatile and oxygen heterocyclic fractions and enantiomeric distribution of volatile components. Journal of Separation Science. 2010;**33**:3374-3385

[4] Cosentino S, Tuberoso CIC, Pisano B, Satta M, Mascia V, Arzedi E, et al. *In vitro* antimicrobial activity and chemical composition of Sardinian *Thymus* essential oils. Letters in Applied Microbiology. 2002;**29**:130-135

[5] Ozogul Y, Kuley E, Ucar Y, Ozogul F. Antimicrobial impacts of essential oils on food borne-pathogens. Recent Patents on Food, Nutrition & Agriculture. 2015;7(1):53-61

[6] Singh P, Pandey AK. Prospective of essential oils of the genus *Mentha* as biopesticides: A review. Frontiers in Plant Science. 2018;**9**:1295. DOI: 10.3389/fpls.2018.01295

[7] Cunha JA, Heinzman BM, Baldisserotto B. The effects of essential oils and their major compounds on fish bacterial pathogens—A review. Journal of Applied Microbiology. 2018;**125**:328-344

[8] Mancuso M, Catalfamo M, Laganà P, Rappazzo AC, Raymo V, Zampino D, et al. Screening of antimicrobial activity of citrus essential oils against pathogenic bacteria and *Candida* strains. Flavour and Fragrance Journal. 2019;**34**(3):187-200. DOI: 10.1002/ffj.3491

[9] Bokhari N, Perveen K, Al Khulaifi M, Kumar A, Siddiqui I. *In Vitro* antibacterial activity and chemical composition of essential oil of *Mentha arvensis* Linn. leaves. TEOP. 2016;**19**:907-915

[10] Fair RJ, Yitzhak T. Antibiotics and bacterial resistance in the 21st century. Perspectives in Medicinal Chemistry. 2014;**6**:25-64. DOI: 10.4137/PMC.S14459

[11] Aycan M, Yildiz M, Darcin S, Tunc K, Hos A, Dundar E. Antibacterial Activity of *Mentha pulegium* L. from Turkey. American Journal of Life Sciences. 2015;**3**:383-386. DOI: 10.11648/j.ajls.20150306.11

[12] Mahalakshmi Prya A, Manikandan M, Kalaiselvi G, Arun P, Chinnaswamy P, Selvam K. Screening on antibacterial activity of *Menta piperita* L. Asian Journal of Microbiology, Biotechnology & Environmental Sciences. 2007;**4**:1049-1052

[13] Hiruma CA. Estudo químico e farmacológico do óleo essencial das folhas de Mentha x villosa Hudson [doctoral thesis]. Universidade Federal da Paraíba; 1993

[14] Monte FJQ, Oliveira EF, Braz-Filho R. Triterpenóides pentacíclicos de *Mentha x villosa*: identificação estrutural e atribuição dos deslocamentos químicos dos átomos de hidrogênio e carbono. Quim Nova. 2001;**24**:491-500

[15] Gobert V, Moja S, Colson M, Taberlet P. Hybridization in the section *Mentha* (Lamiaceae) inferred from AFLP markers. American Journal of Botany. 2002;**89**:2017-2023

[16] Lorenzo D, Paz D, Dellacassa E, Davies P, Vila R, Cañigueral S. Essential oils of *Mentha pulegium* and *Mentha rotundifolia* from Uruguay. Brazilian Archives of Biology and Technology. 2002;**45**:519-524

[17] Marchese JA, Broetto F, Ming LC, Goto R, Stefanini MB, Galina A, et al. Perfil dos consumidores de plantas medicinais e condimentares do município de Pato Branco (PR). Horticultura Brasileira. 2005;**22**:332-342

[18] Sartoratto A, Machado ALM, DelarmelinaC, FigueiraGM, DuarteMCT, RehderVL. Compositionandantimicrobial activity of essential oils from aromatic plants used in Brazil. Brazilian Journal of Mricobiology. 2004;**35**:275-280

[19] Bertini LM, Pereira AF, Oliveira CLL, Menezes EA, Morais SM, Cunha FA, et al. Perfil de sensibilidade de bactérias frente a óleos essenciais de algumas plantas do nordeste do Brasil. Infarma. 2005;**17**:80-83

[20] Bieski IG. *Plantas medicinais e aromáticas no sistema único de saúde da região sul de Cuiabá-MT. Monografia*. MG: Universidade Federal de Lavras; 2005. p. 92

[21] Ullah N, Khurram M, Amin MU, Khan TA, Khayyam SU, Khan FA, et al. Impact of geographical locations on *Mentha spicata* antibacterial activities. Journal of Medicinal Plant Research. 2012;**6**:1201-1206

[22] Snoussi M, Noumi E, Trabelsi N, Flamini G, Papetti A, De Feo V. *Mentha spicata* essential oil: Chemical composition, antioxidant and antibacterial activities against planktonic and biofilm cultures of *Vibrio* spp. strains. Molecules. 2015;**20**:14402-14424. DOI: 10.3390/molecules200814402

[23] Heydari F, Saeedi S, Hassanshahian M. Antibacterial activity of *Mentha longifolia* against *Salmonella typhimurium*. Advanced Herbal Medicine. 2015;**1**:42-47

[24] Moghtader Y, Hadi-Khayatnouri N, Abbasi-Maleki S, Moradi-Kor N. Comparison of antibacterial activity of the hydroalcoholic and essential oil of *Mentha pileglum* in vitro condition. In: 1st International Conference on Medicine, Public Health and Biological Sciences (MPHBS). 2016

[25] Sariri R, Razmgar R, Taheri M, Shaigan Z. The synergic antibacterial effect of green tea and *Mentha pegium* extracts. Clinical Biochemistry. 2011;**44**:S230

[26] Taherpour AA, Khaef S, Yari A, Nikeafshar S, Fathi M, Ghambar S. Chemical composition analysis of the essential oil of *Mentha piperita* L. from Kermanshah, Iran by hydrodistillation and HS/SPME methods. Journal of Analytical Science and Technology. 2017;**8**(11):1-6. DOI: 10.1186/s40543-017-0122-0

[27] Lubbe A, Verpoorte R. Cultivation of medicinal and aromatic plants for specialty industrial materials. Industrial Crops and Products. 2011;**34**:785-801. DOI: 10.1016/j.indcrop.2011.01.019

[28] Hussain AI, Anwar F, Nigam P, Ashraf M, Gilani A. Seasonal variation in content, chemical composition and antimicrobial and cytotoxic activities of essential oils from four *Mentha* species. Journal of the Science of Food and Agriculture. 2010;**90**:1827-1836. DOI: 10.1002/jsfa.4021

[29] Rohloff J, Dragland S, Mordal R, Iversen T. Effect of harvest time and drying method on biomass production, essential oil yield, and quality of peppermint (*Mentha* × *piperita* L.). Journal of Agricultural and Food Chemistry. 2005;**53**:4143-4148. DOI: 10.1021/jf047998s

[30] Figueiredo AC, Barroso JG, Pedro LG, Scheffer JC. Factors affecting secondary metabolite production in plants: Volatile components and essential oils. Flavour and Fragrance Journal. 2008;**23**:213-226. DOI: 10.1002/ffj.1875

[31] Soković MD, Vukojević J, Marin PD, Brkić DD, Vajs V, Van Griensven LJ. Chemical composition of essential oils of *Thymus* and *Mentha* species and their antifungal activities. Molecules. 2009;**14**(1):238-249

[32] Saeed K, Pasha I, Bukhari H, Butt MS, Iftikhar T, Shujah-UdDin U. Compositional profiling of *Mentha piperita*. Pakistan Journal of Food Sciences. 2014;**24**(3):151-156

[33] Alankar S. A review on peppermint oil. Asian Journal of Pharmaceutical and Clinical Research. 2009;**2**(2):27-33

[34] Behnam S, Farzaneh M, Ahmadzadeh M, Tehrani AS. Composition and antifungal activity of essential oils of *Mentha piperita* and *Lavendula angustifolia* on post-harvest phytopathogens. Communications in Agricultural and Applied Biological Sciences. 2005;**71**(3 Pt B):1321-1326

[35] Başer K, Kürkçüoğlu M, Demirci B, Özek T, Tarımcılar G. Essential oils of *Mentha* species from Marmara region of Turkey. Journal of Essential Oil Research. 2012;**24**(3):265-272

[36] Yasukawa K, Yamaguchi A, Arita J, Sakurai S, Ikeda A, Takido M. Inhibitory effect of edible plant extracts on 12-otetradecanoylphorbol-13-acetate-induced ear oedema in mice. Phytotherapy Research. 1993;**7**(2):185-189

[37] Chouhan S, Sharma K, Guleria S. Antimicrobial activity of some essential oils—Present status and future perspectives. Medicines (Basel). 2017;**4**(3):58. DOI: 10.3390/medicines4030058

[38] Singh P, Pandey AK. Prospective of essential oils of the genus *Mentha* as biopesticides: A review. Frontiers in Plant Science. 2018;**9**:1295. DOI: 10.3389/fpls.2018.01295

[39] Ultee A, Bennik M, Moezelaar R. The phenolic hydroxyl group of carvacrol is essential for action against the foodborne pathogen *Bacillus cereus*. Applied and Environmental Microbiology. 2002;**68**(4):1561-1568

[40] Balouiri M, Sadiki M, Ibnsouda SK. Methods for in vitro evaluating antimicrobial activity: A review. Journal of Pharmaceutical Analysis. 2016;**6**:71-79

[41] Kubo I, Muroi H, Kubo A. Antibacterial activity of long chain alcohols against *Streptococcus mutans*. Journal of Agricultural and Food Chemistry. 1983;**41**:2447-2450

[42] Weis N. Zur Wirkweise von Terpenoiden auf den Energiestoffwechsel von Bakterien: Wirkung auf respiratorischen Elektronentransport und oxidative Phoshorylierung [dissertation]. Erlangen: Friedrich-Alexander Universitat; 1986

[43] Budzyńska A, Wieckowska-Szakiel M, Kalemba D, Sadowska B, Rózalska B. The optimization of methods utilized for testing the antibacterial activity of essential oils. Medycyna Doświadczalna i Mikrobiologia. 2009;**61**(3):281-287

[44] Remmal A, Bouchikhi B, Rhayour K, et al. Improved method for the determination of antimicrobial activity of essential oils in agar medium. Journal of Essential Oil Research. 1993;**5**:179-184

[45] Hili P, Evans CS, Veness RG. Antimicrobial action of essential oils: The effect of dimethylsulphoxide on

the activity of cinnamon oil. Letters in Applied Microbiology. 1997;**24**:269-275

[46] Hammer KA, Carson CF, Riley TV. Influence of organic matter, cations and surfactants on the antimicrobial activity of *Melaleuca alternifolia* (tea tree) oil in vitro. Journal of Applied Microbiology. 1999;**86**:446-452

[47] Pauli A. Identification strategy of mechanism-based lipophilic antimicrobials. In: Zhu P, editor. New Biocides Development: The Combined Approach of Chemistry and Microbiology (ACS Symposium Series). Corby: Oxford University Press; 2017. pp. 213-268

[48] Clinical and Laboratory Standards Institute. CAP Laboratory Accreditation Program Inspection Checklist. MIC–Microbiology; 2008

[49] Zaidi S, Dahiya P. *In vitro* antimicrobial activity, phytochemical analysis and total phenolic content of essential oil from *Mentha spicata* and *Mentha piperita*. International Food Research Journal. 2015;**22**:2440-2445

[50] Burt S. Essential oils: Their antibacterial properties and potential applications in food—A review. International Journal of Food Microbiology. 2006;**94**:223-253

[51] Tullio V, Nostro A, Mandras N, Dugo P, Banche G, Cannatelli MA, et al. Antifungal activity of essential oils against filamentous fungi determined by broth microdilution and vapour contact methods. Journal of Applied Microbiology. 2007;**102**:1544-1550

[52] Tyagi AK, Malik A. Antimicrobial action of essential oil vapours and negative air ions against *Pseudomonas fluorescens*. International Journal of Food Microbiology. 2010;**143**:205-210

[53] Mondello F, Girolamo A, Scaturro M, Ricci ML. Determination of *Legionella pneumophila* susceptibility to *Melaleuca alternifolia* Cheel (tea tree) oil by an improved broth micro-dilution method under vapour controlled conditions. Journal of Microbiological Methods. 2009;**77**:243-248

[54] Inouye S, Abe S, Yamaguchi H, Asakura M. Comparative study of antimicrobial and cytotoxic effects of selected essential oils by gaseous and solution contacts. International Journal of Aromatherapy. 2003;**13**:33-41

[55] Botz L, Nagy L, Kocsis B. Detection of microbiologically active compounds. In: Nyiredy SZ, editor. Planar Chromatography, A Retrospective View for the Third Millennium. Budapest: Springer; 2001. pp. 489-516

[56] Horváth G, Botz L, Kocsis B, Lemberkovics E, Szabó LG. Antimicrobial natural products and antibiotics detected by direct bioautography using plant pathogenic bacteria. Acta Botanica Hungarica. 2004;**46**:153

[57] Quiroga EN, Sampietro DA, Sgariglia MA, Soberón JR, Vattuone MA. Antimycotic activity of 5'-prenylisoflavanones of the plant *Geoffroea Decorticans*, against Aspergillus species. International Journal of Food Microbiology. 2009;**132**:42

[58] Moreno L, Bello R, Primo-Yufera E. Pharmacological properties of the methanol extract from *Mentha uaveolens Ehrh*. Phytotherapy Research. 2002;**16**:10-13

[59] Iscan G, Kirimer N, Kurkcuoglu M, Baser KHC. Antimicrobial screening of *Mentha piperita* essential oils. Journal of Agricultural and Food Chemistry. 2002;**50**(14):3943-3946

[60] Elsabee MZ, Abdou ES. Chitosan based edible films and coatings: A review. Materials Science and Engineering. 2013;**33**:1819-1841

[61] Peng Y, Li Y. Combined effects of two kinds of essential oils on physical, mechanical and structural properties of chitosan films. Food Hydrocolloids. 2014;**36**:287-293

[62] Akhter R, Masoodi FA, Wani TA, Rather SA. Functional characterization of biopolymer based composite film: Incorporation of natural essential oils and antimicrobial agents. International Journal of Biological Macromolecules. 2019;**137**:1245-1255

[63] Scartazzini L, Tosati JV, Cortez DHC, Rossi MJ, Flôres SH, Hubinger MD, et al. Gelatin edible coatings with mint essential oil (*Mentha arvensis*): Film characterization and antifungal properties. Journal of Food Science and Technology. 2019;**56**(9):4045-4056. DOI: 10.1007/s13197-019-03873-9

[64] Githaiga BM, Gathuru EM, Waithaka PN, Omondi GO. Antifungal effects of essential oils from mint and rosemary on peronospora destructor and *Candida albicans*. Mediterranean Journal of Basic and Applied Sciences. 2018;**2**(4):05-12

[65] Aydın B, Barbas LAL. Sedative and anesthetic properties of essential oils and their active compounds in fish: A review. Aquaculture. 2020;**520**:734999

Chapter 8

Determination of In Vitro Antiprotease, Antimicrobial, and Antibiofilm Activities of *Beta vulgaris* var. cicla against Multidrug-Resistant Strains of *Pseudomonas aeruginosa*

Hayet Edziri, Rim Nasri, Marwa Hamdi and Maha Mastouri

Abstract

Antibiotic resistance of *Pseudomonas aeruginosa* causes many infectious diseases and it is agreat. So, the aim of the present work was to assess the antibacterial, antibiofilm activity of *Beta vulgaris* extracts against resistance bacteria *P. aeruginosa* that were clinically isolated and tested for their antiprotease potential. Result showed that methanol extract exhibited important antiprotease activity against Trypsin, Savinase, and digestive proteases of blue crab with percentage of inhibition of 94.66, 91.39, and 86.41%, respectively. It showed also important antibiofilm activities against multidrug-resistant *P. aeruginosa* with inhibition values upper than 80% with a concentration of 4MIC. Our investigation delivered that *Beta vulgaris* might be possible source of natural antienzymatic, antimicrobial, and antibiofilm agents.

Keywords: *Beta vulgaris*, antibacterial, antibiofilm, antiprotease, multidrug-resistant *P. aeruginosa*

1. Introduction

Many studies have demonstrated that vegetables play a significant role in human nutrition. They reduced risk of many chronic diseases, like diabetes, cardiovascular illnesses, and cancers [1–3] and Alzheimer's diseases [4, 5]. These advantageous properties of vegetables are due to the bioactive compositions known for their important antioxidant activities [6, 7].

Microbial contamination and the resistance of pathogenic bacteria to antibiotics are considered as major problems of public health [1, 8, 9].

Pseudomonas aeruginosa are bacteria that cause nosocomial infections. They are able to be resistant to a great number of antibiotics such as Carbapenems like imipenem [10, 11].

Beta vulgaris L. belongs to the *Amaranthaceae* family. Its juice had important biological properties like as antimicrobial, hemostatic, and anticancer [12, 13]. *Beta vulgaris* is categorized among the best vegetables with important antioxidant activity; in addition, many researches have showed that *Beta vulgaris* extracts had other important activities (anti-inflammatory, antiallergenic, antithrombotic, and anticoagulant) [14, 15].

The objective of this chapter was to investigate the antiprotease, antimicrobial, and antibiofilm activities of *Beta vulgaris var. cicla* against multidrug-resistant strains of *Pseudomonas aeruginosa.*

2. Materials and methods

2.1 Plant material

The fresh beetroots were bought from a market in Sousse (Tunisia) and the roots were identified and a voucher specimen was placed in our laboratory at the Faculty of Pharmacy (Monastir).

2.2 Preparation of aqueous extract of *Beta vulgaris*

About 200 ml of distilled water was added to 50 g of *Beta vulgaris* pieces. Then they were allowed to boil for 30 min. The extract was filtered using a Whatman paper. The filtrate was kept at −25°C.

2.3 Preparation of methanolic extract of *Beta vulgaris*

Beetroots were washed and sliced into small pieces and then 200 ml of methanol was added to 100-g root in brawn bottle for 3 days at room temperature, filtered through Whatman filter paper, and dried with rotavapor. Then the extract was kept at 4°C.

2.4 Total polyphenol content

The total phenolic content was tested by Folin-Ciocalteu method (Edziri et al.) [16]. The total polyphenols content is expressed as mg gallic acid equivalents (GAEs) per g of extract.

2.5 Total flavonoid content

The flavonoids content was tested by the method of Othmana et al. [17]. The result is expressed in mg quercetin equivalents (QEs) per g of extract.

2.6 Total tannin contents

Total tannin content in *Beta vulgaris* extracts was tested by using Folin-Denis reagent [18].

2.7 Total carotenoid content

Total carotenoids content of *Beta vulgaris* was determined by the ARNON method [19].

2.8 Antiprotease activity

The impact of *Beta vulgaris* extracts, at a concentration of 250 μg/ml, on several proteases' activity was evaluated. So, enzymes were pre-incubated with each extract for 30 min at 30°C. Then, the residual enzyme activity was evaluated according to the method of Georgé et al. [20] using casein as a substrate at the optimal pH and temperature for each enzyme: Purafect (pH 10.0; 50°C), Savinase (pH 10.0; 60°C), (pH 8.5; 50°C) and enzyme of blue crab (pH 8.0; 60°C), trypsin and chymotrypsin (pH 8.0; 37°C). The activity of the enzyme assayed in the absence of inhibitors was taken as 100%.

2.9 Antibacterial activity of *Beta vulgaris* extracts

2.9.1 Microdilution assay

Minimum inhibitory concentration (MIC) values were determined by a microdilution method as indicated by Edziri et al. [21]. The MIC was defined as the lowest concentration that inhibits the development of bacteria, after 24 h of incubation [22].

2.9.2 Antimicrobial activity

2.9.2.1 Micro-well determination of MIC and MBC

The minimum inhibitory concentration (MIC) and minimum bactericidal concentration (MBC) were determined for all bacteria tested in this work by a microdilution method as described by [23]. The MIC was distinct as the lowest concentration of the extract to inhibit the development of the bacteria.

2.9.3 Inhibition of biofilm formation

The biofilm inhibition was tested against five multidrug-resistant strains of *Pseudomonas aeruginosa*, by microdilution technique according to Edziri et al. [21].

3. Results and discussion

3.1 Phytochemical screening

The proportions of the phenols, flavonoids, tannins, and carotenoids contents are summarized in **Table 1**. Methanolic extract of *Beta vulgaris* was the richest with phenols, flavonoids, tannins, and carotenoids as shown in **Table 1**.

3.2 Antiprotease, antibacterial and antibiofilm activities

The antiprotease activity of various *Beta vulgaris* extracts was tested at a concentration of 250 μg/ml. **Table 2** demonstrates that all extracts were able to decrease the protease activities by about 51.53–94.66%, suggesting that they were rich sources of the protease inhibitors. In fact, results revealed that the preincubation of Trypsin, Savinase, and digestive proteases of blue crab with methanol extract caused the loss of 94.66, 91.39, and 86.41% of their activity, respectively; however, a decrease of about 89.31 and 91.39% was observed after incubation of this extract with Purafect and chymotrypsin, respectively.

It is interesting to note that the proteolytic activities of Savinase® and Purafect®, commercial microbial proteases, were mostly inhibited by methanol extract by about 91.39 and 89.31%, respectively. In addition, it was efficient to reduce 94.66% of digestive trypsin activity. In addition aqueous extracts exhibit good antiprotease activity.

According to **Table 3**, the values of MIC for two extracts against multidrug-resistant *Pseudomonas aeruginosa* varied between 50 and 100 mg/ml, without difference between the two extracts of *Beta vulgaris*. Furthermore, the MBC values were of 250 mg/ml. The observed activity of *Beta vulgaris* roots may be attributed to the higher content of polyphenols, flavonoids, and tannin, which are known for their important antimicrobial activity.

The two extracts showed important antibiofilm activity (**Figures 1** and **2**). Furthermore, methanolic extract exhibited the greatest antibiofilm property against all resistant strains of PA with inhibition values greater than 80% at the concentration of 4MIC. In addition, aqueous extract inhibited the biofilm formation of PA greater than 50% with 2MIC. We can observe that there is not any difference between the tested strains of PA. Also methanol extract of *Beta*

	Aq	**M**
Total polyphenols (mg GAE/ g) extract	99.47 ± 0.45	134.55 ± 0.6
Total flavonoids (mg EQ/g) extract	1.29 ± 0.50	4.34 ± 0.02
Total tanin content(mg TA/g)	6.15 ± 1.4	7.5 ± 0.5
Carotenoids (mg/100 g FW)	2.1 ± 1.2	2.97 ± 0.4

GAE: gallic acid equivalent, CE: catchin equivalent, TA: tannic acid, Aq: aqueous extract, M: methanol extract.

Table 1.
Phytochemical analysis of Beta vulgaris *var. cicla*.

Enzymes	**M**	**Aq**
Purafect	89.31 ± 1.13	60.70 ± 0.96
Savinase	91.39 ± 1.38	81.07 ± 0.43
Chymotrypsin	65.28 ± 0.47	51.53 ± 0.51
Trypsin	94.66 ± 0.32	87.42 ± 1.55
Digestive proteases of blue crab	86,41 ± 0.34	70.11 ± 0.61

Values are mean ± SD of three replicate analyses, Aq: aqueous extract, M: methanol extract.

Table 2.
Antiprotease activity of Beta vulgaris *L.*

Strains extracts	**P.S1**		**P.S2**		**P.S3**		**P.S4**		**P.S5**	
	MIC	**MBC**	**MIC**	**MBC**	**MIC**	**MBC**	**MIC**	**MBC**	**MIC**	**MBC**
Aq	100	250	100	250	100	250	100	250	100	250
M	50	250	100	250	100	250	100	250	100	250

Aq: aqueous extract, M: methanol extract, MIC and MBC are in mg/ml.

Table 3.
Antipseudomonal activity of Beta vulgaris *extracts.*

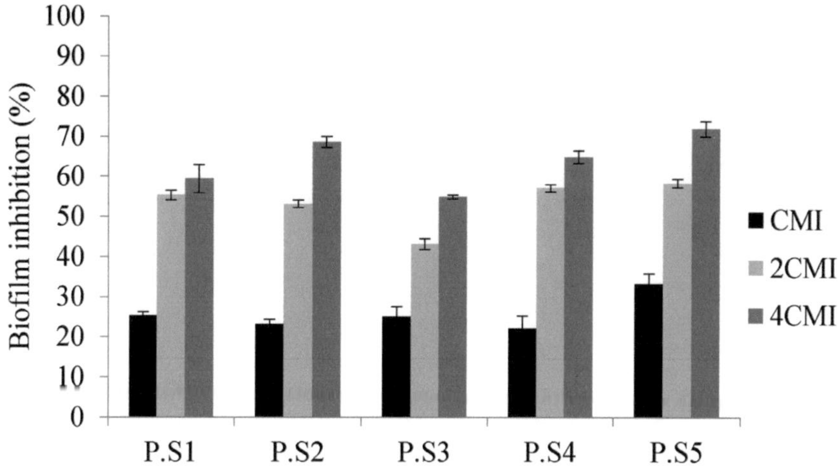

Figure 1.
Antibiofilm activity of Beta vulgaris *aqueous extracts.*

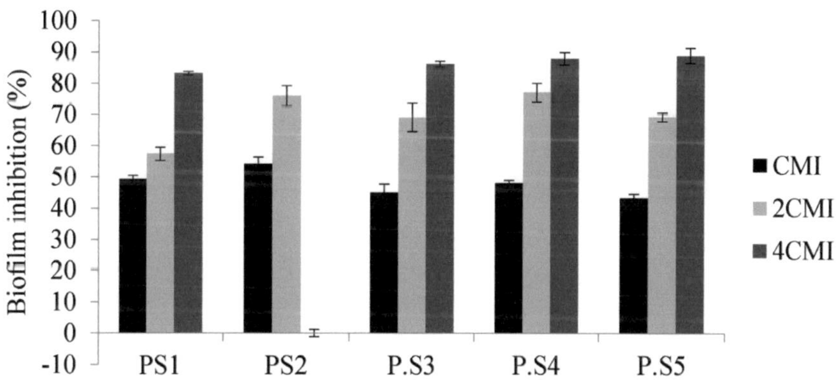

Figure 2.
Antibiofilm activity of Beta vulgaris *methanolic extracts.*

vulgaris displayed a respectable antibiofilm property beside P.S5 with percentages of inhibition of 88.9% at a concentration of 4MIC. The present search was investigated for the first time on the antibiofilm capacity of *Bea vulgaris* against multidrug-resistant strains of *Pseudomonas aeruginosa.* On the other hand, the antibiofilm action is mostly due to the great amount of phenolic content, such as that of flavonoids and tannin known for their good biological activities [24, 25].

4. Conclusion

From this study, we can see that *Beta vulgaris* showed good antiprotease, antibacterial, and antibiofilm activities against different resistant *Pseudomonas aeruginosa* strains. This study also showed that the utilization of this vegetable can lead to the inhibition of bacterial growth.

Furthermore, this vegetable can be used as a source of natural antienzymatic, antimicrobial, and antibiofilm agents. Research is in progress to identify and isolate the bioactive molecules and to test them in vivo.

Author details

Hayet Edziri[1*], Rim Nasri[2], Marwa Hamdi[2] and Maha Mastouri[1]

1 Laboratoire des maladies transmissibles et des substances biologiquement actives, Faculté de Pharmacie, Monastir, Tunisie

2 Laboratory of Enzyme Engineering and Microbiology, National Engineering School of Sfax, University of Sfax, Sfax, Tunisia

*Address all correspondence to: jaziri_hayet@yahoo.fr

References

[1] Wruss J, Waldenberger G, Huemer S, Uygun P, Lanzerstorfer P, Müller U, et al. Compositional characteristics of commercial beetroot products and beetroot juice prepared from seven beetroot varieties grown in Upper Austria. Journal of Food Composition and Analysis. 2015;**42**:46-55

[2] Guldiken B, Toydemir G, Nur Memis K, Okur S, Boyacioglu D, Capanoglu E. Home-processed red beetroot (*Beta vulgaris* L.) products: Changes in antioxidant properties and bioaccessibility. International Journal of Molecular Sciences. 2016;**17**:858

[3] Biondo PBF, Boeing JS, Barizo RO, Souza NED, Matsushita M, Oliveira CCD, et al. Evaluation of beetroot (*Beta vulgaris* L.) leaves during its developmental stages: A chemical composition study. Food Science and Technology (Campinas). 2014;**34**:94-101

[4] Pai SR, D'Mello P. Stability evaluation of beetroot colour in various pharmaceutical matrices. Indian Journal of Pharmaceutical Sciences. 2004;**66**:696-699

[5] Esatbeyoglu T, Wagner AE, Schini-Kerth VB, Rimbach G. Betanin—A food colorant with biological activity. Molecular Nutrition & Food Research. 2015;**59**:36-47

[6] Sainath M, Kumar KS, Babu KA. Formulation and evaluation of herbal lipstic. IJARMPS. 2016;**3**:2058-2060

[7] Vinson JA, Hao Y, Su X, Zubik L. Phenol antioxidant quantity and quality in foods: Vegetables. Journal of Agricultural and Food Chemistry. 1998;**46**:3630-3634

[8] Kähkönen MP, Hopia AI, Vuorela HJ, Rauha JP, Pihlaja K, Kujala TS. Antioxidant activity of plant extracts containing phenolic compounds. Journal of Agricultural and Food Chemistry. 1999;**47**:3954-3962

[9] Vulić J, Čanadanović-Brunet J, Ćetković G, Tumbas V, Djilas S, Četojević-Simin D, et al. Antioxidant and cell growth activities of beet root pomace extracts. Journal of Functional Foods. 2012;**4**:670-678

[10] Ehtesham-Gharaee M, Eshaghi A, Shojaee S, Asili J, Emami SA, Behravan J, et al. Protective effects of *Scutellaria lindbergii* root extract against oxidative-induced cell and DNA damage in mouse fibroblast-like cells. Drug and Chemical Toxicology. 2015;**38**:293-299

[11] Edzir H, Ammar S, Souad L, Mahjoub MA, Mastouri M, Aouni M, et al. *In vitro* evaluation of antimicrobial, antioxidant activities of some Tunisian vegetables. South African Journal of Botany. 2012;**78**:252-256

[12] El-Sabour MF, Abd E-S, Abo MA, Rizk M. Physiological and chemical responses of sunflower to the application of previous organic waste composts to sandy soil. Environmental Management and Health. 1997;**8**:128-132

[13] Ormsbee MJ, Lox J, Arciero PJ. Beetroot juice and exercise performance. Nutrition and Dietary Supplements. 2013;**5**:27-35

[14] Pandey KB, Rizvi SI. Plant polyphenols as dietary antioxidants in human health and disease. Oxidative Medicine and Cellular Longevity. 2009;**2**:270-278

[15] Edziri H, Jaziri R, Chehab H, Verschaeve L, Flamini G, Boujnah D, et al. A comparative study on chemical composition, antibiofilm and biological activities of leaves extracts of four

Tunisian olive cultivars. Heliyon. 2019;**55**:E01604

[16] Saeed N, Khan M, Shabbir M. Antioxidant activity, total phenolic and total flavonoid contents of whole plant extracts *Torilis leptophylla* L. BMC Complementary and Alternative Medicine. 2012;**12**:221

[17] Othmana A, Ismaila A, Ghania NA, Adenan I. Antioxidant capacity and phenolic content of cocoa beans. Food Chemistry. 2007;**100**:1523-1530

[18] Edziri H, Mastouri M, Mahjoub A, Anthonissen R, Mertens B, Cammaerts S, et al. Toxic and mutagenic properties of extracts from Tunisian traditional medicinal plants investigated by the neutral red uptake, VITOTOX and alkaline comet assays. South African Journal of Botany. 2011;**77**:703-710

[19] Jeyanthi RL, Sharmila S, Das MP, Seshiah C. Extraction and purification of carotenoids from vegetables. Journal of Chemical and Pharmaceutical Research. 2014;**6**(4):594-598

[20] Georgé S, Brat P, Alter P, Amiot MJ. Rapid determination of polyphenols and vitamin C in plant-derived products. Journal of Agricultural and Food Chemistry. 2005;**53**:1370-1373

[21] Edziri H, Hechmi A, Chehab H, Luc V, Guido F, Dalenda B, et al. A comparative study on chemical composition, antibiofilm and biological activities of leaves extracts of four Tunisian olive cultivar. Heliyon. 2019;**5**:e01604

[22] Uttara B, Singh AV, Zamboni P, Mahajan RT. Oxidative stress and neurodegenerative diseases: A review of upstream and downstream antioxidant therapeutic options. Current Neuropharmacology. 2009;**7**:65-74

[23] Edziri H, Maha M, Samia A, Mata M, Gros P, Raida H, et al. Antimicrobial, antioxidant, and antiviral activities of *Retama raetam* (Forssk) Webb flowers growing in Tunisia. World Journal of Microbiology and Biotechnology. 2008;**24**:2933-2940

[24] Clark G, Ting KN, Wiart C, Fry J. High correlation of 2,2-diphenyl-1-picrylhydrazyl (DPPH) radical scavenging, ferric reducing activity potential and total phenolics content indicates redundancy in use of all three assays to screen for antioxidant activity of extracts of plants from the Malaysian rainforest. Antioxidants. 2013;**2**:1-10

[25] Dutta-Roy AK, Crosbie L, Gordon MJ. Effect of tomato extract on human platelet aggregation in vitro. Platelets. 2001;**12**:218-227